PREHOSPITAL DRUG THERAPY

SHERYL M. GONSOULIN, BSN, MN

Assistant Professor and Department Head
Emergency Health Science
University of Southwestern Louisiana
Lafayette, Louisiana

WILLIAM RAYNOVICH, NREMT-P, BS, MPH

Director of Prehospital Services
The Reading Hospital and Medical Center
West Reading, Pennsylvania

with **113** *illustrations*

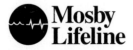
Mosby
Lifeline

St. Louis Baltimore Boston Chicago London Madrid Philadelphia Sydney Toronto

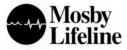

**Mosby
Lifeline**

Dedicated to Publishing Excellence

Executive Editor: Claire Merrick
Developmental Editor: Nancy J. Peterson
Production Editor: Vicki Hoenigke
Senior Book Designer: Gail Morey Hudson
Manufacturing Supervisor: Kathy Grone
Cover illustration: Doug Strutters

Printed in the United States of America

Composition by Mosby Electronic Production, Philadelphia
Printing/binding by R. R. Donnelley & Sons

Mosby–Year Book, Inc.
11830 Westline Industrial Drive
St. Louis, Missouri 63146

Library of Congress Cataloging in Publication Data
Gonsoulin, Sheryl M.
    Prehospital drug therapy / Sheryl Gonsoulin, William Raynovich.
        p.   cm.
    Includes bibliographical references and index.
    ISBN 0-8016-1969-6
    1. Pharmacology.   2. Allied health personnel.   3. Medical
emergencies—Chemotherapy.   I. Raynovich, William.   II. Title.
    [DNLM: 1. Drug Therapy.   2. Emergencies.   WB 105 G639p 1994]
RM301.G65   1994
615.5'8—dc20
DNLM/DCL   93-120
for Library of Congress   CIP

94   95   96   97   98   /DC   9   8   7   6   5   4   3   2   1

Foreword

The importance of safe and knowledgeable drug administration by the paramedic cannot be overemphasized. Throughout my many years of teaching paramedic courses, I have used several books in search of the perfect text to support the pharmacology component of the paramedic curriculum. I believe my search is over.

The ideal text should provide information that is technically accurate and up-to-date, and be specifically applicable to the paramedic. It should be well-illustrated to enhance the reader's understanding. *Prehospital Drug Therapy* provides these features plus, as we say here, *lagniappe*—something extra! Unlike other prehospital pharmacology texts, this book contains learning objectives for each chapter, case presentations to illustrate major principles, and a chapter on pain management. The text is comprehensive in its scope and is very readable.

Prehospital advanced life support is dynamic and requires continued learning and review. This text not only supplies the paramedic student with all of the information necessary for developing a strong knowledge base in pharmacology, but may also serve as an excellent reference text for practicing paramedics.

Ray A. Bias, RN, BSN, CEN, NREMT-P

Director, Medical Resources Department
Acadian Ambulance Service, Inc.
Lafayette, Louisiana

- CDR, NC, USNR
  Commanding Officer, Naval Reserve
  Naval Hospital; Pensacola, Florida—Detachment 210

- EMS Magazine/Braun Industries
  1992 Paramedic of the Year

- Immediate Past Chairman and Member,
  Board of Directors National Registry of EMTs

- Treasurer, Joint Review Committee
  for the Accreditation of EMT-Paramedic programs

Preface

After teaching the pharmacology component of the paramedic curriculum for several years, using a number of paramedic and pharmacology texts, the authors perceived a strong need for a different kind of textbook. *Prehospital Drug Therapy* has been written specifically for the paramedic student. It provides a comprehensive approach to the study of pharmacology. More important, it is directly applicable to prehospital care.

The continual proliferation of new drugs and new information related to drug therapy is staggering. No single textbook, no matter how well written or well researched, can provide everything one needs to know about pharmacology. This book is intended to provide a solid understanding of the principles and practices that support safe and knowledgeable medication administration.

The book is organized into 14 chapters. The first six provide the conceptual basis for understanding specific drug groups and their applications in the field. These chapters include a relevant discussion of the roles and responsibilities associated with drug therapy, a clear presentation of concepts that guide all drug administration, and a comprehensive explanation of dosage calculation and techniques of drug administration.

The remaining eight chapters cover specific emergencies for which drugs are administered. These chapters address drug therapy using a problem-oriented approach. Case studies are used to illustrate the appropriate use of drugs in the prehospital setting.

Specific information about each drug (e.g., indications, precautions, dosages, administration methods) is presented in a drug profile at the end of the chapter to which it relates. Drugs mentioned in one chapter, but profiled in another, are cross-referenced by page number, making the information easily accessible. Further, boxes at the beginning of these chapters list the drugs profiled, their classifications, and the page numbers of their profiles. This format also makes the text useful as a quick reference guide. To get the most value from the text, the student should read each of the drug profiles.

There are other unique features of the text that warrant mentioning. First, the authors had the distinct advantage of completing the manuscript just after the recommendations of the 1992 Conference on Cardiopulmonary Resuscitation and Emergency Cardiac Care were published. All information on the drugs used in advanced cardiac life support reflect the new guidelines. Issues and concerns related to pregnancy, the elderly, and pediatrics are integrated throughout the text. Finally, all information is written at a level appropriate for paramedics and paramedic students, and is specifically relevant to prehospital care.

Sheryl M. Gonsoulin
William Raynovich

Author Acknowledgments

The authors wish to express their appreciation to the many people who have assisted in the writing of this book. We would like to acknowledge Melanie Meche for her numerous contributions to the preparation of the manuscript and her willingness to work at odd hours with pressing deadlines. We would also like to thank Lydia Thibodeaux for her assistance with permission letters and various charts and tables.

We especially want to acknowledge Richard K. Walker, EMT-P, for his contribution to the original text for Chapter 9 and his assistance through the numerous drafts of that chapter. Cynthia A. Phillips, EMT-P, assisted in the writing of the second and final drafts of Chapters 11 through 14. We wish to thank Mark Kirk, MD, who worked closely with the authors in the writing of Chapter 7, and Joseph Thek, MD, for his assistance with Chapter 10. We wish to acknowledge Donovan Grettner, the Public Relations and Marketing Supervisor of Acadian Ambulance Services, Inc., for his photographic skill and endless patience in assisting with the illustration program.

Sheryl Gonsoulin personally thanks Thomas Hernandez, MD, who taught her graduate-level pharmacology course and inspired her love for the subject. His careful review of the early drafts of the first nine chapters of this text is greatly appreciated.

We would also like to thank the reviewers of the text. Their expertise and honest criticism helped enormously in improving the quality of this book. Finally, we would like to thank Nancy Peterson, Claire Merrick, and the staff at Mosby–Year Book for their patience and guidance in bringing this project to completion.

Publisher Acknowledgments

The editors wish to acknowledge the reviewers of this book for their invaluable help in developing and fine-tuning the manuscript, namely:

Mark A. Kirk, M.D.
Assistant Director, Division of Toxicology
Department of Emergency Medicine
Carolinas Medical Center
Charlotte, North Carolina

Janet M. Spellman, BSN, MS, CEN, EMT-P
Assistant Program Director
EMT-Paramedic Program
Northeastern University
Burlington, Massachusetts

Kevin G. Madigan
Critical Care Flight Paramedic
Air Ambulance Programme
Sunnybrook Health Science Centre
Toronto, Ontario, Canada

S. Rutherfoord Rose, Pharm.D., ABAT
Director, Carolinas Poison Center
Instructor, Department of Emergency Medicine
Carolinas Medical Center
Charlotte, North Carolina

Shawn Pruchnicki, R.Ph., BS, EMT-P
Certified Specialist in Poison Information/Education
Central Ohio Poison Control Center
Children's Hospital, Columbus, Ohio
Firefighter/Paramedic
Jackson Township Fire Department
Grove City, Ohio

Anthony S. Manoguerra, Pharm.D.
Director, San Diego Regional Poison Center
University of California San Diego Medical Center
San Diego, California
Professor of Clinical Pharmacy
School of Pharmacy
University of California San Francisco, San Diego Program

Judith A. Cremeens, RN, M.Ed., CEN, NREMT-P
Associate Professor of Emergency Medical Care
Department of Medical Services Technology
Eastern Kentucky University
Staff Nurse, Emergency Department
Pattie A. Clay Hospital
Richmond, Kentucky

We also thank Diane Lofshult for lending us her editorial expertise, and Dwight Polk, EMT-P, for his review of artwork.

A Note to the Reader

Every attempt has been made to provide information that is consistent with widely accepted standards and current medical literature. Because the science of pharmacology is continually advancing, our knowledge base continues to expand. Therefore, we recommend that the reader always check product information for changes in dosage and administration before administering any medication. The drugs presented in this book should only be administered by direct order, either verbally or through accepted standing orders, of a licensed physician.

Any procedure described in this book should be applied by the readers in accordance with professional standards and local protocol as defined by their medical directors. The authors and publisher disclaim any liability for the consequences of the use and application of any of the contents of this book.

Contents

1

Introduction to Prehospital Drug Therapy

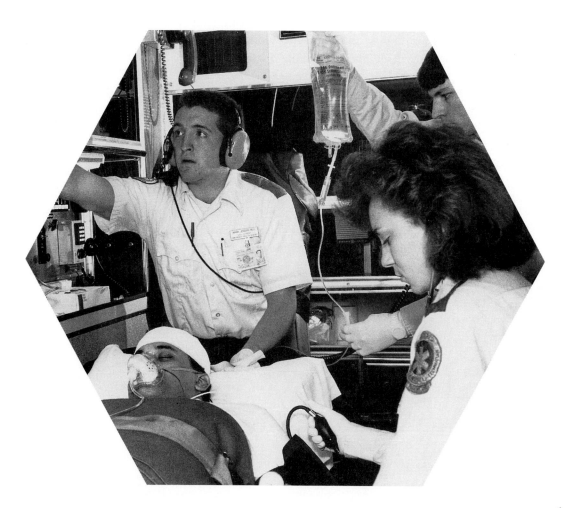

OBJECTIVES

1. Define pharmacology.
2. Explain the paramedic's responsibilities related to prehospital drug therapy.
3. List four sources from which drugs are derived.
4. Differentiate the chemical, generic, and trade names of drugs.
5. Compare sources of drug information.

A **drug** is broadly defined as any chemical that affects living processes. The study of drugs and their actions on living systems is referred to as **pharmacology**. Drug therapy is broader in scope than pharmacology in that drug therapy encompasses not only knowledge of drug action and interaction but also information related to drug administration, patient assessment, and clinical judgment.

The administration of drugs is an area of prehospital care that distinguishes advanced life support providers from basic life support providers. Maintaining current knowledge and skills related to drug therapy is not an easy task, given the dynamic nature of emergency medicine. New drugs are continually being introduced, and new information is continually being discovered about existing drugs.

Paramedics should develop an understanding of the concepts and principles underlying drug therapy to guide their practice. Such an understanding enables paramedics to recall the details of drug actions and side effects as part of a predictable pattern instead of simply memorizing specific facts about specific drugs.

The purpose of this text is to provide paramedic students with the information essential to ensure the safe and effective administration of drugs in the prehospital setting. This chapter addresses the historical evolution of drug therapy, drug legislation, roles and responsibilities of the paramedic, drug sources, drug nomenclature, and sources of drug information.

KEY TERMS

Drug—any chemical that affects living processes.
Pharmacology—study of drugs and their interactions with living systems.

HISTORICAL PERSPECTIVE

The use of drugs to treat pain and illness dates to antiquity. Primitive people were attended by medicine men who subjected the sick to mysterious rites and a large collection of crude preparations. The Ebers Papyrus, writings that contain information on ancient Egyptian pharmacology and medicine, lists remedies such as oil, wine, yeast, turpentine, gums, resins, opium, iron, lead, and soda. The therapeutic effects of such remedies were largely derived by trial and error.[3]

An example of a primitive drug that was used effectively is purple foxglove. Its use as a diuretic was first described in 1250 A.D. as a treatment for "dropsy" (an outdated term used to describe generalized edema). It was not until approximately 1800 that the effect of purple foxglove on the heart was first described. Digitalis, the active ingredient in purple foxglove, is still a commonly prescribed cardiac drug.

Although the discovery of penicillin was somewhat accidental, the antibiotics of the 1930s and 1940s represent some of the most significant medical advances of all times. Before the discovery of these agents, physicians could do little to treat infections.[3]

In contrast to earlier times, today's new drugs are usually the result of well-developed, scientific studies. There are literally thousands of drugs on the market today with a wide variety of therapeutic uses. Many of these drugs have implications for use in the emergency setting.

DRUG LEGISLATION

The current regulation of the manufacture and sale of drugs in the United States is extensive. Organizations involved in regulating the manufacture and sale of drugs are listed in Table 1-1. The federal Food and Drug Administration (FDA) is responsible for the approval of drugs before they are made available for general use in the United States. The FDA enforces compliance with standards established by various acts of legislation. Although such regulation has on occasion caused delays in the release of potentially beneficial medicines, it has for the most part ensured the availability of safer and more effective drugs. In spite of extensive regulation, however, adverse reactions or complications of drug therapy are sometimes not detected until the drug has been in use.

The Pure Food and Drug Act of 1906 was the first law enacted in the United States to regulate drugs. This law provided for the establishment of the FDA, required drugs to be free of adulterants or contaminants, and prohibited the sale of medicinal preparations that had little or no use. The law

Table 1-1 Organizations Involved in Regulating the Manufacture and Sale of Drugs in the United States

NAME	COMMON ACRONYM	FUNCTION
Department of Health and Human Services (formerly Department of Health, Education, and Welfare)	HHS	The secretary of HHS is a cabinet-level officer whose duties include designating the official names for drugs sold in the United States and overseeing the Public Health Service.
Drug Enforcement Administration	DEA	This agency within the Department of Justice is the sole drug enforcement arm of the U.S. government, under the Controlled Substances Act of 1970.
Federal Trade Commission	FTC	This federal agency regulates the advertisement of medications aimed at the general public (not medical personnel).
Food and Drug Administration	FDA	This federal agency is responsible for guaranteeing the safety, purity, effectiveness, and reliability of drugs sold in the United States. In addition, this agency regulates the advertising of medications to medical personnel.
National Academy of Sciences–National Research Council	NAS–NRC	The NAS is a private organization composed of outstanding scientists in the United States. The NRC is the research arm of NAS and was involved in evaluating the efficacy of drugs for the FDA in the Drug Efficacy Study Implementation.
Public Health Service	PHS	This federal agency not only funds extensive clinical research but also is responsible for maintaining basic research programs under the National Institutes of Health. Biologicals used as drugs are also certified by this agency.
Pharmaceutical Manufacturers Association	PMA	This private organization represents the pharmaceutical houses where most drugs are developed. This group functions as an advisory group to the FDA on occasion and as a lobbying group to Congress.
United States Adopted Names Council	USAN	This private group contains members from government, private industry, the medical profession, and research institutions whose function is to advise the Secretary of HHS as to the appropriate official name for each new drug introduced.

From Clark JB, Queener SF, Karb VB: *Pharmacological basis of nursing practice*, ed 4, St Louis, 1993, Mosby–Year Book.

Table 1-2 Important Drug Legislation (United States)

Food, Drug and Cosmetic Act of 1938	Mandated that drug manufacturers must test all drugs for harmful effects and that drug labels must be accurate and complete
Wheeler-Lea Act of 1938	Defined criteria for nonfraudulent advertising
Durkham-Humphrey Amendment of 1952	Distinguished more clearly between drugs that can be sold with or without a prescription and those that cannot be refilled
Drug Amendment of 1962 (Kefauver-Harris Act)	Tightened controls over drug safety and statements about adverse reactions and contraindications; drug testing methods; and drug effectiveness criteria
Controlled Substances Act of 1970 (Comprehensive Drug Abuse Prevention Act of 1970)	Categorized controlled substances based on their relative potential for abuse
Drug Regulation Reform Act of 1978	Shortened the drug investigation process to release drugs sooner to the public

From McKenry LM, Salerno E: *Mosby's pharmacology in nursing*, ed 18, St Louis, 1992, Mosby–Year Book.

was inadequate because it did not address drug safety or effectiveness. Numerous other legislative acts have since been passed that more effectively control the manufacture and sale of drugs in the United States (Table 1-2).

In 1970 the Comprehensive Drug Abuse Prevention and Control Act, commonly referred to as the Controlled Substances Act, was passed. This act established rules for the manufacture and distribution of drugs considered to have potential for abuse. The law provided that such drugs be classified into five categories referred to as *schedules*. Table 1-3 provides characteristics, dispensing restrictions, and examples of each of these schedules.

The Controlled Substances Act requires accurate accounting for the use of scheduled drugs. All agencies that administer scheduled drugs are required by law to adhere to specific policies related to the record keeping and disposal of unused portions of controlled substances. Examples of scheduled drugs that are commonly administered in the prehospital setting are meperidine and morphine sulfate (Schedule II) and diazepam (Schedule IV).

ROLES AND RESPONSIBILITIES

The safe and timely administration of the correct drug can make the difference between life and death in serious emergencies. In less dramatic circumstances drug administration can provide increased comfort, relief of

Table 1-3 Schedule of Controlled Substances

SCHEDULE	CHARACTERISTICS	DISPENSING RESTRICTIONS	EXAMPLES (PARTIAL LIST)
I	High abuse potential No accepted medical use—for research, analysis, or instruction only May lead to severe dependence	Approved protocol necessary	Heroin, marijuana (cannabis), tetrahydrocannabinols, LSD, mescaline, peyote, psilocybin, methaqualone
II	High abuse potential Accepted medical uses May lead to severe physical and/or psychologic dependence	Written Rx necessary (signed by the practitioner)—only emergency dispensing permitted without written Rx (only required amount may be prescribed for emergency period) No Rx refills allowed Container must have warning label*	Opium, morphine, hydromorphone, meperidine, codeine, oxycodone, methadone, secobarbital, pentobarbital, amphetamine, methylphenidate, cocaine, and others
III	Less abuse potential than drugs in Schedules I and II Accepted medical uses May lead to moderate/low physical dependence or high psychologic dependence	Written or oral Rx required Rx expires in 6 months No more than 5 Rx refills allowed within a 6-month period Container must have warning label*	Preparations containing limited quantities of, or combined with, one or more active ingredients that are noncontrolled substances: codeine, hydrocodone, morphine, dihydrocodeine or ethylmorphine, and nonnarcotic drugs such as derivatives of barbituric acid except those that are listed in another schedule, glutethimide, methyprylon, chlorphentermine, paregoric, and others
IV	Lower abuse potential compared with Schedule III Accepted medical uses May lead to limited physical or psychologic dependence	Written or oral Rx required Rx expires in 6 months with no more than 5 Rx refills allowed Container must have warning label*	Barbital, phenobarbital, chloral hydrate, meprobamate, fenfluramine, chlordiazepoxide, diazepam, oxazepam, clorazepate, flurazepam, lorazepam, dextropropoxyphene, pentazocine, mazindol, alprazolam, and others

Courtesy Winthrop Laboratories, New York, NY. Modified from Ruggieri NL: *Drug Therapy,* 10(12):58-64, 1980, and the DEA pharmacist's manual—an informational outline of the Controlled Substances Act of 1970, US Dept of Justice, Washington, DC, June 1980. (Data apply to federal CSA and Uniform Controlled Substances Act; state laws may differ.)
*Caution: Federal laws prohibit the transfer of this drug to any person other than the patient for whom it was prescribed.

Table 1-3   Schedule of Controlled Substances—cont'd

SCHEDULE	CHARACTERISTICS	DISPENSING RESTRICTIONS	EXAMPLES (PARTIAL LIST)
V	Low abuse potential compared with Schedule IV Accepted medical uses May lead to limited physical or psychologic dependence	May require written Rx or be sold without Rx (check state law)	Medications, generally for relief of coughs or diarrhea, containing limited quantities of certain opioid controlled substances

From Clark JB, Queener SF, Karb VB: *Pharmaceutical basis of nursing practice*, ed 4, St Louis, 1993, Mosby–Year Book.

Table 1-4   Medications Carried by Advanced Life Support Services in the United States (The Percentages Represent the Percentage of Services Surveyed that Carry the Medications Listed in Each Column)

≤1%	≤10%	≤25%	≤50%	≤75%	100%
Alutane	Heparin	Meperidine	D_5W-0.45NS	Verapamil*	Ringer's lactate*
Amyl nitrate	MgSO$_4$*	Nubaine	Glucagon*	Activated	0.9 NS*†
Tigan	Phenytoin	Plasmalyte	Metaproterenol	charcoal	D_5W*†
Calcium	Metaraminol	Albuterol*	Oxytocin*	CaCl$_2$*	Dopamine*†
gluconate	Phenobarbital	D_5W-RL	Procainamide*†	Aminophylline*	Epinephrine*†
Proparicaine	Haloperidol	Digoxin	Thiamine*		Furosemide*
Alucain	Hydroxyzine	Isoetherine	Terbutaline		Diazepam*†
Apomorphine	Phenergan	Nitroglycerin			Morphine SO$_4$*
Apresoline	Acetaminophen	paste			Ipecac
Pancuronium	Methylprednisolone	Nitroglycerin			Isoproterenol*†
Alteplase	Dobutamine	spray			Lidocaine*†
Methergine	Mannitol*	Nifedipine			Naloxone*
Labetalol	Physostigmine	Nitrous oxide			Nitroglycerin
Midazolam	Norepinephrine	Propranolol			SL*†
Hespan	Albumin				NaHCO$_3$*†
D_5W-0.2 NS					Atropine†
Succinylcholine					D_{50}W
Butorphanol					Bretylium†
Hydrocortisone					
Nitroglycerin					
(IV)					
Isosorbide					
dinitrate					
Vecuronium					
D_{10}W					
D_5NS					

From Lavery RF et al: A survey of advanced life support practices in the United States, *Prehosp Disast Med* 7(2):145, 1992.
D_5W, Dextrose 5% in water; D_{10}W, Dextrose 10% in water; D_{50}W, Dextrose 50% in water; NS, Normal saline; D_5NS, Dextrose 5% in normal saline.
*The American Heart Association Advanced Cardiac Life Support Drugs.
†The American College of Emergency Physicians Suggested Drugs.

pain, and other therapeutic benefits to patients in the prehospital setting. Conversely, the wrong drug, dose, or method of administration can harm a patient or even result in death. It is imperative, then, that paramedics have a strong foundation in the principles of pharmacology, develop safe practices related to drug administration, and familiarize themselves with drugs commonly used in the prehospital setting.

Paramedics *administer* drugs under the order of physicians, as only licensed physicians can *prescribe* drugs. Orders for drugs may be communicated directly to paramedics via radio or cellular telephone by a physician or other designated emergency personnel. This practice is referred to as *on-line medical direction.* In some circumstances, written standing orders, or **protocols**, are used by paramedics. Such *off-line* medical direction is usually reserved for life-threatening emergencies in which contact with medical direction would delay treatment or for situations in which communication with medical direction is not possible.

Drugs administered by paramedics vary from state to state and sometimes from county to county within a state. Although the paramedic's scope of practice is most often legislated by the state, many states have provisions for local medical authority to determine specifically which drugs may be given in the prehospital setting. *It is the responsibility of the individual paramedic to be familiar with local protocol and state law.*

A recent study of 170 urban emergency medical services (EMS) in the United States indicated that more than 80 different medications were carried in varying combinations (Table 1-4).[4] The survey showed that the medications recommended by the American Heart Association Advanced Cardiac Life Support guidelines were carried by almost every service. Drugs recommended by the American College of Emergency Physicians, however, were carried less frequently. It was found that, of the services surveyed, the hospital-based services carried the most medications, whereas fire department services carried the fewest.[4]

DRUG SOURCES

Drugs are derived from four main sources: plants, animals, minerals, and laboratory synthesis. From the beginning of time, plants have been the major source of drugs. Before laboratory processing became a standard part of drug

---

KEY TERMS

Protocols—specified treatment regimens; standing orders; a set of procedures to be followed under specific circumstances.

manufacturing, people would chew on leaves or stems or swallow plant seeds to achieve a desired therapeutic effect. Unfortunately, in this crude form, doses and their resulting effects varied greatly and were difficult to predict. When the active ingredient of a drug is separated from its crude form and purified, the refined drug is more concentrated and more predictable in terms of its action.

Certain drugs, such as those used in the treatment of pain, cardiac care, and chemotherapy, continue to be derived from plant sources. However, most drugs previously derived from plants are synthetically manufactured today. Materials such as oils, gums, and resins obtained from plants are also used as components of medications.

Drugs derived from animal sources are also widely used. Probably the most widely used of these drugs is insulin, which has traditionally been derived from bovine or porcine pancreatic tissue. Other drugs obtained from animal sources include epinephrine, corticosteroids, and various hormones. Like drugs derived from plant sources, pure animal derivations are also being replaced by laboratory-synthesized substances, such as synthetic hormones. Additionally, mineral sources provide a number of drugs (e.g., iron, potassium, and calcium preparations).

DRUG NOMENCLATURE

As new drugs are developed they are assigned as many as three names. The first name assigned during the initial investigative stage is the drug's **chemical** name. The chemical name is an exact description of the chemical composition and molecular structure of the drug. Chemical names are generally only used by chemists and pharmacologists during the preliminary stages of drug development. For this reason this text will not cite the chemical names of the drugs discussed.

The **generic** name, which is assigned and approved by the United States Adopted Name Council, is the official name of the drug in the United States. The generic name of a drug is often related to the chemical name in some way and is completely independent of the drug's manufacturer(s).

The **trade** name (also called brand name or proprietary name) is designated by the specific manufacturer of a drug. A drug may have several trade names but only one generic name. Unfortunately, having several trade names for the same drug can prove confusing for patients. They may duplicate their medications by assuming that different trade names signify different drugs. Table 1-5 lists the chemical, generic, and trade names of several commonly used medications. *Note that trade names are capitalized whereas generic names are not.*

Table 1-5 Examples of Drug Names

TRADE	GENERIC	CHEMICAL
Ecotrin, Empirin, Aspergum, Ascriptin	Aspirin	Acetylsalicylic acid
Tempra, Tylenol, Liquiprin	Acetaminophen	N-acetyl-para-amino-phenol
Dilantin	Phenytoin sodium	Diphenylhydantoin sodium
Isuprel	Isoproterenol hydrochloride	Isopropylarterenol, Isopropylnorodrenaline, Isopropylnorepinephrine

Paramedics and other health-care professionals should use generic names to prevent confusion. However, there are a number of drugs used in prehospital care that are commonly referred to by their trade name by physicians and paramedics (e.g., Narcan, Valium, and Lasix). This textbook cites the generic name and common trade names when a drug is introduced; thereafter the generic name is used.

SOURCES OF DRUG INFORMATION

The *United States Pharmacopeia* and the *National Formulary* are two publications that contain all the drugs and formulations officially approved by the FDA. More practical sources of drug information are the *American Hospital Formulary Service*, published by the American Society of Hospital Pharmacists, and the *AMA Drug Evaluation*, prepared by the American Medical Association Department of Drugs. Both of these publications are periodically revised and updated. A more widely used but less complete source of drug information is the *Physician's Desk Reference* (PDR). The PDR is a compilation of manufacturers' package inserts.

For the paramedic, more practical "handbooks" are indicated for quick, accurate information on emergency drugs. As a result of the ever-increasing number of drugs used in the field, it is unrealistic to expect paramedics to recall in-depth information pertinent to all emergency drugs. Reference handbooks have, therefore, become a necessary part of the paramedic's equipment. However, for students, textbooks are generally the most appropriate source of drug information because they describe groups of drugs in relation to their therapeutic uses and provide other information necessary for beginners.

SUMMARY

Pharmacology is the study of drugs and their interaction with living systems. The regulation of the sale and manufacturing of drugs in the United States is controlled by numerous organizations and legislative acts.

Drugs are derived from animal, plant, mineral, or synthetic sources. Drugs receive several names during their development. The generic name is the official name of a drug; trade names are the names given a drug by a specific manufacturer. Chemical names are complex and rarely used by health-care professionals. Paramedics refer to medications by either their generic or trade name.

Paramedics administer drugs under the order of a physician. Although the paramedic's scope of practice, including drug administration, is usually legislated at the state level, many states have provisions for local medical authorities to determine which drugs should be given in local EMS services. It is an individual's responsibility to be familiar with local protocol and state law.

To provide safe and effective drug therapy paramedics must be familiar with prehospital drug indications, contraindications, actions, therapeutic effects, side effects, routes and rates of administration, and potential interaction with other drugs the patient has taken. It is difficult for paramedics to remember all the necessary relevant information about every drug they administer. However, numerous resources for drug information are available to paramedics.

REFERENCES

1. Garrison HG et al: Paramedic skills and medications: practice options utilized by local advanced life support medical directors, *Prehosp Disast Med* 6(1):29, 1991.
2. Gilman AG et al: *Goodman and Gilman's pharmacological basis of therapeutics*, ed 8, New York, 1990, Pergamon Press.
3. Hernandez T: *Know your medicine*, New York, 1990, Carlton Press.
4. Lavery RF et al: A survey of advanced life support practices in the United States, *Prehosp Disast Med* 7(2), 1992.
5. Pepe PE: The past, present, and future of emergency medical services, *Prehosp Disast Med* 4:47, July-September 1989.
6. Pepe PE: Regulating the scope of EMS services, *Prehosp Disast Med* 5(1):59, 1990.
7. Shuster M, Chong J: Pharmacologic interventions in prehospital care: a critical appraisal, *Ann Emerg Med* 18:192, 1989.
8. Smith JP, Bodai BI: The urban paramedics scope of practice, *JAMA* 253:544, 1985.

2

Drug Action and Interaction

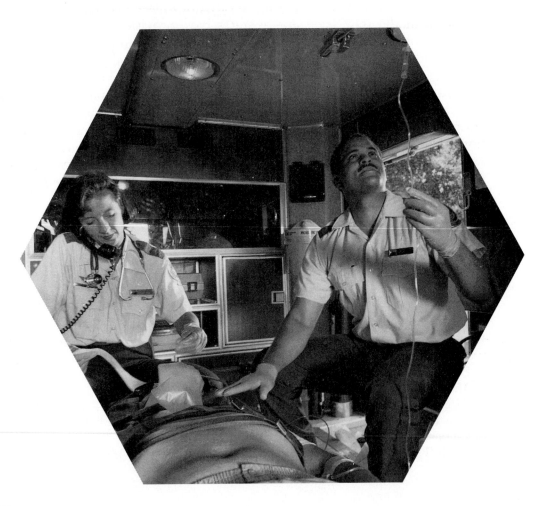

OBJECTIVES

1. Define pharmacokinetics and pharmacodynamics.
2. Discuss factors that affect drug absorption.
3. Explain how cardiovascular function affects the distribution of a drug.
4. Identify factors that influence the rate and efficiency of drug metabolism.
5. List the primary organs for drug excretion.
6. Explain three ways in which a drug may exert its action on tissues.
7. Identify factors that determine where and how a drug will act in the body.
8. List two types of synergistic drug effects.
9. Identify three mechanisms of antagonistic drug interaction.
10. Describe characteristics of pediatric and geriatric patients that influence drug distribution, metabolism, and excretion.

As the number of drugs used in emergency medicine has grown, so have the responsibilities and the level of knowledge required of paramedics. To provide optimal care paramedics must possess knowledge about all aspects of drug therapy, not only regarding routine doses and routes of administration but also as to how drugs work and why they are administered.

This chapter presents information fundamental to the knowledgeable administration of emergency drugs. **Pharmacokinetics** and **pharmacodynamics** are the major concepts addressed in this chapter.

PHARMACOKINETICS

Simply stated, pharmacokinetics is the study of the fate of drugs in the body (Figure 2-1). Pharmacokinetics refers to how drugs enter the body (**absorption**), how they reach their site of action (**distribution**), how they are transformed (**metabolism** or **biotransformation**), and how they are removed from the body (**excretion** or **elimination**).

KEY TERMS

Pharmacokinetics—fate of drugs in the body, including absorption, distribution, metabolism, and excretion.

Pharmacodynamics—study of the way drugs act on living tissues.

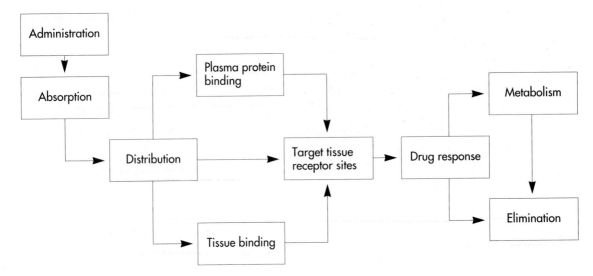

Figure 2-1   Fate of a drug from administration to elimination.

Each drug has its own characteristic rate of absorption, distribution, metabolism, and excretion. The intensity of a drug's action is influenced by the concentration of the drug in the plasma at any given time (see box on page 15).

Absorption

Absorption is the process by which a drug moves from its site of entry into the body fluid that will carry it to its site of action. The rate of absorption determines how quickly a drug becomes available to exert its action. With the exception of direct intravenous (IV) administration, all routes of drug administration require that some degree of absorption take place. Because IV administration introduces the drug directly into the circulation, the need for absorption is negated. Factors that influence drug absorption include solubility, **pH**, site of absorption, and circulation to the site of administration.

Solubility. Solubility refers to the process by which the solid form of a drug dissolves in the body fluids. Oral forms of solid drugs should be administered with plenty of fluids because drugs must be in solution before they can be absorbed from the gastrointestinal tract into the blood. Although oral medications are rarely used in the field, it is important that paramedics have a basic understanding of the principles of absorption. Many patients take oral medications that have implications for prehospital care.

PLASMA LEVEL TERMS

Loading dose: Initial dose of a drug given in sufficient amount to achieve a therapeutic plasma level

Maintenance dose: Dose of a drug necessary to maintain a constant therapeutic plasma concentration

Onset of action: Time interval between the administration of a drug and the first sign of its effect; onset of action is influenced by the physical and chemical properties of a drug as well as by its route of administration

Plasma (serum) level: Amount of the drug present in plasma; peak level refers to the highest concentration produced by a specific dose

Therapeutic range: Difference between the minimal therapeutic and toxic concentrations of a drug; drugs with a low therapeutic range present a higher risk of toxicity than drugs with a high therapeutic range; also referred to as the margin of safety

Toxic level: Plasma concentration at which severe adverse reactions are expected

Toxicity: Degree to which a substance is poisonous; drugs can produce toxic effects at high doses that are not seen at lower doses

pH. The **pH** of a drug refers to how *acidic* or *alkalinic* (basic) the drug is. The pH of a drug and the pH of the drug's environment can affect the rate at which the drug diffuses across the cell membrane. An acidic drug readily diffuses across the membranes and into the circulation in an acidic environment. For example, aspirin, an acidic drug, readily diffuses across the cell membranes into circulation in the stomach's acidic environment. If the pH of the drug is altered (e.g., as with buffered aspirin) or the pH of the stomach is altered (e.g., through antacid ingestion), drug absorption is slowed. The opposite is true of drugs in a basic environment; basic drugs are easily absorbed, whereas acidic drugs are not.

Site of absorption. Drug molecules pass through a single layer of cells (e.g., intestinal epithelium) much more readily than through multiple layers, such as skin. Therefore absorption from the gastrointestinal tract generally occurs more rapidly than across the skin (**transdermal**). However, when slow, prolonged absorption is desired, the transdermal route is ideal. The size of the absorbing surface also affects the absorption rate. Generally, the larger the surface, the more quickly a drug is absorbed. For example, inhaled drugs are quickly absorbed from the pulmonary epithelium as a result of its very large surface area.

Circulation. Generally, drugs administered in sites with a rich blood supply (**sublingual**) are absorbed much more quickly than those administered in a poorly vascularized site, such as subcutaneous tissue. Also, systemic blood flow can affect the rate at which a drug is absorbed from a site. For example, drugs given orally, subcutaneously, or intramuscularly to patients in shock may be poorly and unreliably absorbed. This is why intravenous administration is most often indicated in emergency situations.

Distribution

Distribution is the process by which a drug is carried from the site of absorption to the site of action. Once a drug enters the bloodstream it is distributed throughout the body and ultimately to its site of action. Factors that influence distribution are cardiovascular function, drug storage reservoirs, and physiologic barriers.

Drug distribution is impaired in any situation in which cardiac output is decreased, such as with shock and congestive heart failure. Cardiac output dramatically affects the rate of distribution, and regional variations in blood flow also affect distribution rates. Organs with extensive blood supply, such as the heart and kidneys, receive drugs more quickly than areas with less extensive blood supply, such as the muscles and skin.

Drug storage reservoirs can also influence the distribution of a drug. Storage reservoirs exist in two forms: plasma protein binding and tissue binding. The physical-chemical properties of a drug will determine its **binding capacity**.

On entry into systemic circulation, many drugs attach to plasma proteins, particularly albumin, to form a drug-protein complex. Because this drug-protein complex is too large to diffuse across membranes, bound drugs are pharmacologically inactive until released from the binding site. Only the free, unbound portion of a drug can act on a **target site**. As an unbound drug is metabolized a portion of the bound drug is released, thus prolonging the duration of the action.

The degree to which a drug is bound to plasma protein is generally expressed as a percentage. For example, propranolol is normally 90% protein bound, which means that, at any given time, 10% of that drug is free to act, whereas 90% is bound to plasma protein. **Toxicity** can result if this

---

KEY TERMS

Binding capacity—degree to which a drug is bound to tissue or plasma proteins at any given time.

Toxicity—degree to which a substance produces undesirable or harmful effects.

ratio is disturbed. Factors that can disturb this ratio are decreased levels of plasma protein and the concurrent administration of another highly protein-bound drug. Hypoalbuminemia, a condition that is characterized by low serum albumin levels, decreases the number of binding sites and results in a higher level of unbound drug available for distribution to target tissues. Concurrent administration of a second highly bound drug results in competition for binding sites, leading to displacement of the first drug. Again, this results in a higher level of unbound drug available for distribution to target tissues.

Tissue binding occurs in fat and bone tissue. Lipid-soluble drugs have a high **affinity** for fat tissue and become stored and concentrated in fat. Because blood flow is relatively low in fat tissue, drugs stored in this area are not quickly distributed. If another dose of the drug is given too soon, the additional amount is also stored in the fat tissue. This may result in a **cumulative effect**. Additionally, there may be a prolonged action even after the drug is discontinued. An example of a lipid-soluble drug is diazepam (Valium). In addition to its affinity for fat tissue, diazepam is highly protein-bound. This results in an extremely long **half-life** and a prolonged period of drug action.

Physiologic barriers also influence the distribution of a drug. The blood-brain barrier is a physiologic barrier that serves to protect brain tissue from exposure to certain substances. The blood-brain barrier is highly selective, preventing the passage of many drugs into the brain. This barrier causes most drugs to be absorbed more slowly by the brain than by other tissues. For example, epinephrine, when injected intravenously, exerts significantly less effect on the central nervous system than on the peripheral nervous system.

Metabolism

Most drugs undergo metabolism, or biotransformation, a process by which drugs are inactivated and converted into a product that can be elimi-

---

KEY TERMS

Cumulative effect—drug effects that develop when a dose is repeated before a prior dose is metabolized; drugs are accumulated and eventually produce symptoms of toxicity.

Half-life—amount of time required to reduce the concentration of a drug in the blood by 50%; the amount of time required for 50% of a drug to be eliminated from the body; half-life does not change with drug dose.

nated from the body. The primary site of metabolism is the liver, but other tissues, such as plasma, kidneys, lungs, and intestinal mucosa, may also be involved in this process.

Several factors influence the rate and efficiency of drug metabolism. People with impaired cardiac function, liver disease, or kidney disease frequently have prolonged drug metabolism. Drug metabolism is also affected to some degree by the genetic makeup of an individual. Infants and older adults also experience depressed drug metabolism. In the infant this is a result of immaturity of the liver and kidneys during the first few months of life. Degenerating metabolizing enzyme systems, chronic disease, and less efficient renal function depress metabolism in the elderly. Ultimately, delayed or depressed drug metabolism can result in prolonged response to a drug or in cumulative effects when multiple doses are given. It should be noted that metabolism does not always lead to the formation of "less active" compounds. It can cause the formation of equally active products (as with ephedrine) or even more toxic products (as with lidocaine) than the original drug.

Excretion

The kidneys are the primary organ of excretion for drugs or inactive drug metabolites. The next most common site for drug excretion is the intestines. Drugs may also be excreted from the body by the lungs, the skin, and the sweat, salivary, and mammary glands.

PHARMACODYNAMICS

Pharmacodynamics is the study of the effect of drugs on living tissues. In effect, pharmacodynamics answers the question, "How does this drug work, and why am I giving it?" A drug's **mechanism of action** is the way in which it produces a desired effect. Most drugs exert their mechanism of action in one of the following ways:

1. Drug-receptor interaction: Some drugs have a special affinity for a certain part of the cell wall or a special site within the cell to produce its effect. This is the most common mechanism of action.
2. Drug-enzyme interaction: Some drugs exert their effect by acting on the enzyme system of a cell.
3. Nonspecific drug interaction: Many drugs have a nonspecific receptor site or site of action. Their therapeutic effect is more generalized, such as in the alteration of the chemical composition of body fluid seen with sodium bicarbonate administration.

The interactive relationship between drugs and receptor sites is frequently compared to that of a lock and key (Figure 2-2). The drug is the key that must fit into the lock or receptor to elicit a response. The ability of the drug to fit the receptor site is dependent on its chemical structure. The ability of a drug to elicit a biologic response is referred to as the drug's efficacy.

Agonists are drugs that cause a change in cellular function when inserted into a receptor site. Receptors may also be occupied by drugs called antagonists. When a drug is an antagonist, the chemical code is similar enough to fit into the receptor but not exact enough to elicit a specific response. An antagonist may have a higher affinity for a receptor site than the agonist, thereby blocking the action of the agonist.

Where and how a drug acts in the body is determined by two factors: (1) localization of receptors, and (2) concentration of the drug to which the receptor is exposed. Localization refers to specific receptors confined to certain locations in the body.

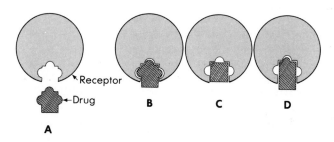

Figure 2-2 **A,** Drugs act by forming a chemical bond with specific receptor sites, similar to a key and lock. **B,** The better the "fit," the better the response. Those with complete attachment and response are called "agonists." **C,** Drugs that attach but do not elicit a response are called "antagonists." **D,** Drugs that attach, elicit a small response, but also block other responses, are called "partial agonists." (From Clayton PD, Stock YN: *Basic pharmacology for nurses*, 9th ed, St Louis, 1989, Mosby–Year Book.)

DRUG RESPONSE TERMS

Adverse reactions: Development of undesirable and potentially harmful side effects

Habituation: Psychological or emotional dependence on a drug after repeated use

Hypersensitivity: Exaggerated response to a drug, usually idiosyncratic in origin

Idiosyncrasy: Abnormal, unpredictable response to a drug peculiar to an individual

Side effect: Effect of a drug other than that which is desired

Tolerance: Decreased response to a drug with repeated doses

Drugs can elicit a variety of responses when administered (see box on page 19). When a drug interacts with specific receptors that are unique to specialized cells, its effects are specific. Conversely, if the drug acts by interacting with nonspecific receptors that are common to most cells, its effects are more widespread, or nonspecific. Although no drug ever produces one single effect, those drugs that act on specific receptors usually produce fewer side effects.

For example, epinephrine may be given to patients with asthma, for the treatment of bronchospasm. While epinephrine acts therapeutically to dilate the bronchioles, thereby improving ventilation, it also acts on other systems, causing increased heart rate, renal artery vasoconstriction, and increased myocardial oxygen consumption. Terbutaline is more selective than epinephrine for specific receptor sites and provides the same therapeutic outcome but with fewer and less dangerous side effects.

Drug Interaction

Drug interaction refers to the process through which the expected therapeutic effect of a drug is altered by the introduction of another factor, usually another drug or chemical agent. When two or more drugs are given simultaneously, they may act to either enhance or diminish the action of the other, or they can produce toxic reactions.

The combined effects of two or more drugs are generally either synergistic or antagonistic. **Synergism** is an enhanced response resulting from concurrent use of two or more drugs. Two types of synergistic effects are:
1. Additive effect: The sum of the effects of two drugs (1 + 1 = 2).
2. Potentiation: The net response of two drugs is greater than the individual effect of either drug if given alone. The combined effect of the two drugs is greater than simple addition (1 + 1 = 3 or more).

Antagonistic interactions occur when one drug interferes with and either reduces or negates the effect of another. Three mechanisms of **antagonism** are:
1. Competition: Drugs compete for the same receptor sites (e.g., narcotic analgesics and naloxone (Narcan), which is a narcotic antagonist).
2. Chemical: The introduction of the second drug causes inactivation of the first by forming a chemical complex.
3. Physiologic: The biologic responses to two drugs are opposite (e.g., barbiturates and amphetamines).

Not all drug interactions are harmful or even undesirable. Indeed, some drug interactions are planned for their desired effects. For example, the beta-blocker propranolol may be given concurrently with a diuretic to potentiate the antihypertensive effect. Narcotic analgesics are often given in combination with other drugs for additive or potentiative effects. An important therapeutic antagonism is the action of naloxone, a narcotic antagonist, which is used to treat narcotic overdose.

AGE-RELATED CONSIDERATIONS

Age is an important factor in the body's response to drugs. The very young and very old are at a higher risk for adverse effects to drugs than older children and younger adults. Also, many precautions must be taken when administering drugs to women of childbearing age. These issues are discussed in the following sections.

Pediatric Patients

Approximately 75% of the drugs marketed in the United States have no established pediatric dose. Therefore pediatric drug doses are usually prescribed according to body weight or body surface area and follow current recommendations from the American Academy of Pediatrics and the American Heart Association. It is vital, therefore that paramedics determine the mass, or body weight, of the child as soon as possible. Although parents are usually the most reliable and quickest sources of such information, they are not always available in emergencies. Paramedics must then estimate the body weight as accurately as possible.

Neonates (birth to 4 weeks of age) are at extremely high risk for adverse drug effects. Their liver and renal functions are not well-developed at this stage, which results in impaired drug metabolism and excretion.

Geriatric Patients

People over the age of 65 currently compose almost 12% of our population, and this number is growing.[4] Like pediatric patients, the elderly have less effective protective mechanisms than younger adults and are at greater risk for accidental trauma. As society ages, geriatric patients will compose a large percentage of the calls answered by an emergency medical services system.

Most experts divide the elderly into the "young old" and the "old old." The purpose of this division is to emphasize that aging adults are not all the same, either physiologically or emotionally. However, as the aging process continues, physiologic and emotional changes become more pronounced.

In addition to the normal physiologic changes of aging the elderly have an increased incidence of illness. Normal physiologic changes include decreased circulating blood volume, which causes drugs to have higher circulating concentrations, and decreased serum albumin for binding, which leads to more free drug in the circulation. Also, decreased renal and liver function cause higher concentrations of drugs as a result of diminished rates of metabolism and excretion. Common illnesses that are prevalent among the elderly population, such as congestive heart failure, can further impair cardiac, renal, and liver function.

Adverse effects of all drugs can be pronounced in the elderly. Elderly patients generally require smaller doses of drugs than younger adults. Particular caution must be taken with drugs that cause side effects of hypotension, as the hypotension produced in the elderly can progress to shock. Antiarrhythmic drugs are particularly notorious for producing drastic side effects in the elderly. For example, lidocaine, when not effectively metabolized, produces symptoms of confusion, delirium, hypotension, and further dysrhythmias. Lidocaine doses and rates of administration should be cut in half for patients over age 65.

Beta-blockers are another group of drugs that cause serious effects in the elderly. The hypotensive effects of beta-blockers may be perilous, and the hypothermic effects associated with beta-blockers leave the older adult susceptible to hypothermia.

All of this translates to one simple fact for the emergency-medical care provider: a large portion of patients you come in contact with will be elderly, and most elderly patients will already be on one or more maintenance drugs. When combined with drugs administered in emergencies, the possibilities for adverse drug reactions are staggering. For this reason it is important to obtain a thorough history of the patient, including present prescription and nonprescription medications the patient is taking.

WOMEN OF CHILDBEARING AGE

When administering drugs to a woman of childbearing age, paramedics should determine whether the patient is pregnant. Any agent that is ingested, inhaled, or absorbed by the mother has the potential to harm the fetus. The Federal Drug Administration categorizes drugs according to their safety in pregnancy (see box on page 23). Drugs should be given only when their potential benefit outweighs the risk of receiving the drug.

During pregnancy, protein binding is decreased and metabolism in the liver is delayed. The rate of drug excretion may be increased because of the increased cardiac output that occurs in pregnancy.

FDA PREGNANCY SAFETY CATEGORIES

Category A

Studies indicate no risk to fetus.

Category B

Animal reproductive studies indicate no risk to the fetus; adequate and well-controlled studies in pregnant women are unavailable.

Category C

Animal reproductive studies indicate an adverse effect on the fetus, but adequate and well-controlled studies in pregnant women are not available. Potential benefit to risk must be evaluated, as it may be warranted to use drug in selected pregnant women at risk.

Category D

Human data or studies exhibit positive evidence of human fetal risk, but potential benefit to risk may warrant the use of the drug in pregnant women.

Category X

Fetal abnormalities and positive evidence of fetal risk in humans are available from animal or human studies or from marketing reports. The risks of using this drug far outweigh the benefits; thus such drugs should not be used in pregnant women.

From McKenry LM, Salerno E: *Mosby's pharmacology in nursing*, ed 18, St Louis, 1992, Mosby–Year Book.

The rate and degree to which a drug crosses the placenta is determined by the specific chemical makeup of the drug. Examples of prehospital drugs that rapidly cross the placenta are lidocaine, meperidine, propranolol, and diazepam.

SUMMARY

A basic understanding of pharmacokinetics and pharmacodynamics is fundamental to the administration of emergency drugs. A knowledge of pharmacokinetics, the study of the fate of drugs in the body, provides paramedics with the understanding of how drugs are absorbed, distributed, metabolized, and excreted. Drug absorption and distribution can be affected by the route of administration, the physical characteristics of the drug, and the blood flow in and around the site of absorption and target tissues. Drug metabolism and excretion are depressed in the very young and very old and in certain conditions.

Drugs produce their mechanism of action in several ways: by acting on a certain part of the cell membrane, by acting on the enzyme system of a cell, or by generalized, nonspecific effects, such as alteration in pH of a body fluid.

REFERENCES

1. Gilman AG et al: *Goodman and Gilman's pharmacological basis of therapeutics*, ed 8, New York, 1990, Pergamon Press.
2. Jones SA et al: *Advanced emergency care for paramedic practice*, Philadelphia, 1992, JB Lippincott.
3. McKenry LM and Salerno E: *Pharmacology in nursing*, ed 18, St Louis, 1992, Mosby–Year Book.
4. Samuels D: Emphasizing the elderly in the new EMT curriculum, *J EMS* 16(6):44, 1991.

3

Safety in Drug Administration

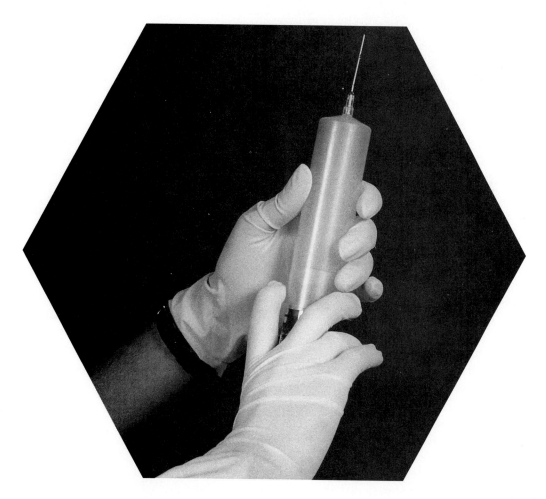

OBJECTIVES

1. Explain the five rights of drug administration.
2. Discuss the advantages of enteral and parenteral drug administration.
3. Differentiate among oral, sublingual, and buccal administration of drugs.
4. Describe the technique for administering drugs via an endotracheal tube.
5. Discuss the safe handling and disposal of sharps in the prehospital setting.
6. Compare intradermal, subcutaneous, and intramuscular injection techniques.
7. Identify appropriate landmarks, and locate injection sites for deltoid, vastus lateralis, rectus femoris, ventrogluteal, and dorsogluteal sites.
8. Describe the technique for deltoid, vastus lateralis, rectus femoris, ventrogluteal, and dorsogluteal intramuscular injections.
9. List reasons for initiating IV therapy.
10. Compare various types of IV administration sets.
11. Describe two types of IV catheters and needles.
12. Discuss criteria for selecting a vein for IV therapy.
13. Explain the technique for initiating IV therapy.
14. Discuss potential complications of IV therapy.
15. Explain the technique for IV push drug administration.
16. Discuss intraosseous medication administration in the prehospital setting.

Prehospital emergency care inevitably involves high-stress situations with intense pressure to perform procedures quickly. Often numerous people other than the paramedic crew are present at emergency scenes, including nonmedical emergency responders, family members, and bystanders. Resources for consultation are typically limited, and multiple tasks must be performed, some simultaneously.

Because of these distractions, limitations, and constraints, it is imperative that paramedics develop safe habits, discipline, and a solid knowledge base of pharmacology and drug therapy. Even in emergencies, with all of the accompanying disorder, patients have the right to safe drug therapy.

This chapter discusses (1) procedures and practices for the safe administration of drugs in the field, (2) drug forms, (3) routes of drug administration, and (4) techniques of drug administration. Although this chapter emphasizes safety in prehospital drug therapy, most paramedic students learn to give medication in the hospital. Thus a number of important differences between the two settings are addressed.

PRINCIPLES AND PRACTICES FOR SAFE ADMINISTRATION OF MEDICATIONS

Verification of the Medical Order

Paramedics have many responsibilities related to drug administration. Initially, they are responsible for assessing, interpreting, and relaying pertinent information regarding the patient's condition to medical direction so that decisions related to the need for medication can be made and an appropriate order given.

Medication orders are typically stated by giving the name of the drug, the dose desired, the route of administration, and when appropriate, the rate (e.g., "Give morphine sulfate, 2 mg, IV push, over two minutes."). Ideally, it is best to write the order down as it is received. However, writing the order is not always possible in the field. Once the physician gives an order the paramedic has the responsibility to verify it by restating the order indicating the drug, the dose, and the route. This ensures that the order was heard correctly. The order should be restated once more to the crew immediately before administering it to the patient (e.g., "I'm giving 2 mg of morphine sulfate IV push.").

Paramedics must evaluate the appropriateness of orders as they are received. Should the dose ordered or potential side effects be of concern, the order must be clarified with medical direction prior to administering the drug. When a paramedic is concerned that an order for a medication is incorrect, local guidelines must be followed. However, the general procedure to follow is to first discuss the concerns with medical direction as the order is given, and if the physician reaffirms the order after being questioned, paramedics must follow the order. If, however, the paramedic is certain that giving the drug will harm the patient, he must notify the physician that he intends to withhold giving the drug and state why he intends to do so. It is important to realize that should the administration of a drug directly harm the patient, the paramedic will be held liable along with the physician.

Sometimes an unusually large or small dose of a drug may be ordered, which differs from local protocols. An example is an order for atropine to be given to a patient with organophosphate poisoning. The maximum dose of atropine typically stated by local emergency medical services (EMS) protocols is 2 mg. In patients with severe organophosphate poisoning, however, continued administration of atropine may be indicated in doses of 2 mg every 5 minutes. A paramedic who refuses to exceed the protocol and does not administer the prescribed follow-up doses would be responsible for withholding a life-saving drug.

Paramedics must make appropriate judgments when carrying out standing orders or when implementing protocols when on-line medical direction is unavailable.

Five Rights of Drug Administration

Once a medication order has been verified, drugs should be given in accordance with the five rights of drug administration: the right patient, the right drug, the right time, the right dose, and the right route.

The right patient. Ensuring that the patient is the right one is a much more common problem in the hospital than in the prehospital setting. However, drug orders have been given and received for the wrong patient in the field. Mistakes occur when paramedics recontact medical direction for additional orders and information updates, and the physician confuses the patient with another who has a similar condition but is with another similarly designated unit (e.g., two "Medic One" units from different parts of a county). Communication difficulties in multiple-casualty incidents also sometimes lead to patient identification confusion (i.e., a situation in which there may be several "chest injuries"). Patient identification confusion can also occur when several units with similar designations or names are calling for patient orders simultaneously. Instances of overcrowded radio frequencies have caused orders for patients to be confused. Unfortunately, there are no simple precautions to ensure that such confusion does not occur. The best safeguard is the knowledgeable paramedic who recognizes an incorrect order and questions the medical director.

The problem of ensuring that the patient is the right one is more common in the hospital where there are many more patients in a unit and patients are constantly being admitted, discharged, and moved from room to room. When a drug is administered in the hospital, the correct safety procedure is to identify the patient through three different methods: (1) asking the patient his or her name (e.g., "What is your name?," not, "Are you Mr. Smith?"); (2) checking the patient's identification bracelet; and (3) checking the name on the door or wherever the patient's name is located in the room.

The right drug. To ensure that the right drug is given the drug label should be read carefully each time a drug is administered. Paramedics develop a certain familiarity with the arrangement of drugs in their drug boxes. Most can open the box and place their hands directly on the medication needed. Such familiarity should not cause paramedics to become complacent about reading labels.

Paramedics must be very cautious when checking the packaging of each drug. For example, lidocaine is packaged in 100 mg doses for intravenous (IV) bolus administration, and 1 g packages for IV infusion. The color, size, and print on the packages are nearly identical, especially at 0300 hours in a dimly lit room. Drugs that are to be administered by infusion only, however, are packaged in containers with protected administration sites to guard against direct bolus administration.

Paramedics must check drug labels carefully every time they prepare to administer a medication. They must read the label to check the name of the drug, the concentration, and the expiration date. The label should be checked as the medication is removed from the drug box, before the prescribed dose is prepared, and once more just before it is administered to the patient. Although checking the label 3 times may seem impractical in extreme emergencies, it is a time-honored standard that takes only a few seconds to do but prevents serious errors.

Errors in giving the wrong drug can occur when one paramedic receives the order and another prepares the drug for administration. Sometimes a third paramedic is the one to actually administer it. No unlabeled drug should ever be administered unless the paramedic has prepared the drug for administration personally, or unless the drug is handed to the paramedic with the original container at the same time.

The right time. Medication orders in emergency settings are generally **stat** orders. This means the drug is to be given as soon as possible and only once. There are, however, other medications used during emergencies that are repeated at specific time intervals or as the patient's condition warrants. For example, during a cardiac arrest epinephrine is given every 5 minutes. Such time intervals should be adhered to as closely as possible to maintain the desired blood levels of the drug being given.

Also related to the right time of administration is the *rate of administration*, the period of time over which a drug is administered. Many drugs must be given at a very precise rate. Administering these drugs at a faster or slower rate than prescribed can have serious consequences for the patient. For example, the rate of administration for dopamine is usually between 2 and 10 µg/Kg/min, while atropine must be administered rapidly via IV **bolus**. A bolus of dopamine could be instantly lethal to a patient, whereas a slow infusion of atropine may worsen bradycardia, causing a paradoxical slowing of the heart rate.

The right dose. The need for accuracy in drug calculation and preparation (i.e., correctly measuring the dose) is crucial. Most of the drugs used in the prehospital setting are available in single-unit packages, or unit doses, which simplify calculations. Reference charts with precalcu-

---

KEY TERM

Bolus—method of IV medication administration by which a drug is rapidly administered rather than infused over a period of time.

lated flow rates are useful. On the other hand, many of the vasoactive drugs used in advanced life support are given according to body weight and require more complex calculations. It is important that paramedics be familiar with an accurate method of dosage calculation for situations in which more than one unit dose or only a portion of a unit dose is ordered. (Dosage calculation is addressed in Chapter 4.)

It is appropriate for paramedics to use dosage charts when they are readily available. In fact the American Heart Association's Pediatric Advanced Life Support course recommends the use of dosage charts for pediatric emergencies because of the wide range of doses for children of differing ages and sizes. Traditionally, paramedics have committed to memory adult doses used in Advanced Cardiac Life Support. It is still advisable, however, for protocols or algorithms to be easily accessible rather than relying totally on memory. Although the dose is determined by medical direction, paramedics need to be familiar enough with the drugs they administer to recognize a questionable dosage. The reference charts used on EMS units and those used by medical direction should be identical.

It is safer when medical direction orders the administration of a drug to be infused in drops per minute (gtts/min). Medical direction typically has more time to compute flow rates under less pressure than paramedics at the scene. This does not, however, relieve paramedics of the responsibility to calculate the correct flow rate quickly and accurately.

The right route. Administering a drug by the wrong route can have serious consequences. Routes are prescribed for specific purposes. For example, epinephrine is given subcutaneously to asthma patients because it is absorbed slowly, providing relief for about 20 minutes. Should epinephrine be given intramuscularly by selecting too long a needle or using an incorrect angle, the patient would not derive the benefits of slower absorption afforded by the subcutaneous route. Similarly, if a drug for relief of pain is administered subcutaneously when ordered intramuscularly, the patient's relief will be delayed.

Documentation

Accurate and thorough documentation is critical in drug administration, both clinically and legally. The following information should be recorded on the paramedic's run report: name of the drug, dosage, route, time, site of administration, and signature of the person administering the drug. In the event an ordered drug is not given the order should be recorded and the reasons why the drug was not given should be documented.

ROUTES OF ADMINISTRATION

As discussed in Chapter 2, the route of administration of a drug ultimately affects the rate and extent of drug absorption. The remainder of this chapter discusses the various routes of administration and drug forms, and describes the techniques for administration and injection of drugs via each of the major routes.

Enteral

Enteral administration refers to drugs administered along any part of the gastrointestinal tract, including the **sublingual, buccal, rectal, and oral routes.** Oral administration is the safest and easiest route of drug administration and is by far the most common route used in the hospital setting and at home. It is rarely used in prehospital care, however, because of its slow rate of absorption. The time it takes an orally administered drug to be absorbed often exceeds the time it takes to transport the patient to the hospital. Also, oral medications are usually administered with water. In patients with an altered level of consciousness, a compromised airway, or a potential need for an emergency surgical procedure, oral intake is contraindicated. Although infrequent, there may be situations in which paramedics are required to administer enteral forms of drugs.

Parenteral

Parenteral administration refers to drugs that are given by injection. The following routes are classified as parenteral: **intradermal, in which the** drug is injected just below the epidermis; **subcutaneous (SC), in which the** drug is injected into the tissue below the dermal layer; **intramuscular (IM),** in which the drug is injected into the skeletal muscle; **intravenous, in which** the drug is injected directly into the circulatory system via a superficial or central vein; **intraosseous (IO), in which the drug is injected into the** medullary canal of a long bone; **endotracheal, in which the drug is instilled** into the trachea via an endotracheal tube; and **inhalation, in which the drug** is inhaled in the form of a fine mist or gas.

Parenteral routes of administration are used by paramedics far more frequently than enteral routes for several reasons. Parenteral absorption is significantly more reliable than enteral absorption because drugs administered parenterally are not affected by factors such as gastric pH or the amount of food that has been ingested. Parenteral absorption is also generally faster than enteral, thereby affording a faster therapeutic effect for the patient. Table 3-1 compares absorption rates of all pertinent routes of drug administration.

Table 3-1 Summary of Major Routes for Systemic Administration of Drugs

ROUTE	DESCRIPTION	ADVANTAGES	DISADVANTAGES
Oral	Drug swallowed, absorbed from stomach and/or small intestine	1. Convenient 2. Nonsterile procedure 3. Economical	1. Unpleasant taste may cause patient to discontinue medication 2. Irritation to gastric mucosa may induce vomiting 3. Patient must be conscious 4. Drug may be partly or completely destroyed by digestive juices 5. Absorbed drug enters portal circulation to liver, where drug may be destroyed.
Sublingual	Drug dissolved under tongue; absorbed across mucous membranes of mouth	1. Convenient 2. Nonsterile procedure 3. Drug enters general circulation before passing through liver	1. Route is not useful for drugs that taste bad 2. Irritation to oral mucosa may occur 3. Patient must be conscious 4. Only very lipid-soluble drugs are absorbed rapidly enough to be administered by this route
Buccal	Drug dissolved between cheek and gum; absorbed across mucous membrane of mouth	As for sublingual	As for sublingual
Transdermal	Drug absorbed directly through skin	1. Continous dosage 2. Nonsterile 3. Drug enters general circulation before passing through liver	1. Effective only for lipid-soluble drugs 2. Local irritation can occur 3. Discarded patches may pose danger of poisoning
Rectal	Drug inserted into rectum; absorbed through mucous membranes of rectum	1. May be used in unconscious or vomiting patient 2. Drug enters general circulation before passing through the liver	1. Route is inconvenient 2. Drug may irritate rectal mucosa 3. Drug must be made up into suppository
Inhalation	Drug inhaled as gas or aerosol	Useful for drugs intended to act directly on lung Useful for drugs that are gases at room temperature and very lipid soluble (i.e., inhalation anesthetics)	Inhalation of lung mucosa may occur

From Clark JB, Queener SF, Karb VB: *Pharmacological basis of nursing practice*, ed 4, St Louis, 1993, Mosby–Year Book.

Table 3-1 Summary of Major Routes for Systemic Administration of Drugs—cont'd

ROUTE	DESCRIPTION	ADVANTAGES	DISADVANTAGES
Subcutaneous	Drug injected under skin	1. Useful for drugs in soluble or relatively insoluble forms 2. May be used in unconscious or uncooperative patients	1. Sterile procedures are necessary 2. Route produces relatively painful site, and patient may suffer irritation from drug
Intramuscular	Drug injected into muscle mass	1. Relatively rapid absorption, since blood supply is good 2. Useful for drugs in soluble or relatively insoluble forms 3. May be used in unconscious or uncooperative patients	1. Sterile procedures are necessary 2. Minor pain is present on injection for most drugs, but irritation and local reaction may occur
Intravenous	Drug injected directly into vein	1. Allows direct control of blood concentration of drug 2. Most rapid attainment of effective blood levels	1. Sterile procedures are necessary 2. Too rapid injection may produce transient, dangerously high blood concentrations of drug

Although parenteral drug administration is invaluable in the prehospital setting, there are disadvantages or risks of which paramedics must be keenly aware. First, the drug administered parenterally bypasses all the body's natural defense mechanisms. Thus there is a greater risk of infection because the natural barriers of the skin and enteric tract are bypassed. Many ingested toxins induce vomiting, which is also a natural defensive process. Another disadvantage with parenteral administration is that **injected or inhaled drugs cannot be retrieved.** Therefore paramedics must be absolutely certain that the parenterally administered drug is the correct medication at the correct dose.

DRUG FORMS

Drugs are supplied in many different forms: capsules, tablets, suspensions, and elixirs are a few examples. Generally, a drug form is *route-specific,* meaning the drug is manufactured in a form that is meant to be administered for a specific route.

Certain drugs, however, are supplied in several different forms. For example, theophylline, a drug commonly used for respiratory problems, is supplied in several forms for oral dosage alone: uncoated tablets for rapid gastrointestinal absorption, enteric-coated tablets for delayed absorption, extended-release capsules for sustained blood levels, and oral liquids. In

Table 3-2 Forms of Medications

FORM	DESCRIPTION
Capsules	Solid dosage forms for oral use in which medication is enclosed in gelatin shell that dissolves in stomach or intestine. Gelatin of capsules is colored to aid in product identification. Various manufacturers use distinctive shapes for distinguishing their capsules from those of other companies.
Douche	Aqueous solution used as cleansing or antiseptic agent for part of body or body cavity. Douches are usually sold as powder or liquid concentrate to be dissolved or diluted before use.
Elixirs	Clear fluids designed for oral use and containing primarily water and alcohol with glycerin and sorbitol or another sweetener sometimes added. Alcohol content of these preparations varies.
Glycerites	Solutions of drugs in glycerin; they are primarily for external use. Solution must be at least 50% glycerin.
Patches	The inner surface of the patch contacts the skin and allows transdermal absorption of relatively lipid-soluble drugs. The total amount of drug in the patch is very large, but typically only a small fraction is absorbed.
Pills	Solid dosage forms for oral use in which drug and various vehicles are formed into small globules, ovoid, or oblong shapes. True pills are rarely used; most have been replaced by compressed tablets.
Solution	Liquid preparations, usually in water, containing one or more dissolved compounds. Solutions for oral use may contain flavoring and coloring agents. Solutions for intravenous injection must be sterile and particle free. Other injectable solutions must be sterile. Solutions of certain drugs may also be used externally.
Suppositories	Solid dosage forms to be inserted into body cavity where medication is released as solid melts or dissolves. Suppositories frequently contain cocoa butter (cacao butter or theobroma oil), which is solid at room temperature but liquid at body temperature, or glycerin, polyethylene glycol, or gelatin, which dissolves in secretions from mucous membranes.
Suspension	Finely divided drug particles that are suspended in suitable liquid medium before being injected or taken orally. Suspensions must not be injected intravenously.
Sustained action	Form of medication that is altered so that dissolution is slow and continuous for extended period. Total dosage in sustained action medication is greater than for regular formulations, since drug is not all released at once but over extended period.
Syrups	Medication dissolved in concentrated solution of sugar such as sucrose. Flavors may be added to mask unpleasant taste of certain medications.

From Clark JB, Queener SF, Karb VB: *Pharmacological basis of nursing practice*, ed 4, St Louis, 1993, Mosby–Year Book.

Table 3-2 Forms of Medications—cont'd

FORM	DESCRIPTION
Tablets	Solid dosage forms, frequently shaped like disks or cylinders, that contain, in addition to drug, one or more of the following ingredients: binder (adhesive substance that allows tablet to stick together), disintegrators (substances promoting tablet dissolution in body fluids), lubricants (required for efficient manufacturing), and fillers (inert ingredients to make tablet size convenient).
Enteric-coated	Solid dosage forms intended for oral use. Medication in tablet form is coated with materials designed not to dissolve in stomach. Coatings do dissolve in intestine, where medications may be absorbed.
Press-coated or layered	Preformed tablet has another layer of material pressed on or around it. This practice allows incompatible ingredients to be separated and causes them to be dissolved at slightly different rates.
Tincture	Alcoholic or water-alcohol solutions of drugs.
Transdermal creams	Relatively lipid-soluble drugs that may be absorbed transdermally. Dosage is usually measured in inches of cream extruded from tube. Protection of the site may be necessary to prevent accidental removal of the cream.
Troches (also called lozenges or pastilles)	Solid dosage forms, frequently shaped like disks or cylinders, that contain drug, flavor, sugar, and mucilage. Troches dissolve or disintegrate in mouth, releasing medication such as antiseptic or anesthetic for action in mouth or throat. Troches dissolve more slowly than tablets.

addition, the drug is supplied in specially prepared liquids as aminophylline for parenteral administration and in suppositories for rectal administration.

It is most important that paramedics carefully read the drug package to determine that the correct preparation is being administered. Even though the right drug is administered, giving the patient the wrong preparation can prove dangerous. An example of this is the frequently used, IV administered antidysrhythmic drug lidocaine, which is also used as a local anesthetic. IV administration of lidocaine intended for use as a local anesthetic can cause serious adverse effects for the patient. Table 3-2 describes the various forms of drug preparations.

TECHNIQUES IN DRUG ADMINISTRATION

Oral

Although oral administration of a drug is a fairly simple process, the following factors must be considered:

1. Aseptic technique should be used as follows:
   a. Wash hands; don gloves.
   b. Tap one dose, typically one pill or capsule, out of the bottle and onto the lid, and then drop it onto the patient's or paramedic's hand for administration.
   c. Don't replace contaminated pills, such as those that have been out of the bottle and on a hand or other surface, back into the original bottle.
2. Oral tablets and capsules should be followed by sufficient fluid intake, usually 4 to 5 oz of water, because a drug must be in solution to be absorbed from the intestine.
3. Ascertain that the patient has actually swallowed the drug. If there is any question, check the area between the patient's cheek and gum and under the tongue for unswallowed medication.
4. Many patients, especially the very young and very old, have difficulty swallowing tablets and capsules. In this situation it is acceptable to either open the capsule or crush the tablet and put it in a little fluid or food to make it easier for the patient to swallow. *Some drugs, however, should not be crushed.* See box below for a list of drugs that should not be crushed.

MEDICATIONS THAT SHOULD NOT BE CRUSHED

The following is a partial listing of drugs that should not be crushed. Whenever possible, it is suggested that if a liquid dosage form of the medication is available, it should be used instead of a crushed tablet. Coated tablets generally should not be crushed because the coating was applied for a specific reason, such as (1) to prevent stomach irritation (e.g., Dulcolax tablets), (2) to prevent destruction by stomach acids (e.g., Ananase), (3) to produce a prolonged or extended effect (e.g. Dimetapp), or (4) to avoid an unwanted reaction (e.g., chloral hydrate in capsule has a very bitter taste and Povan tablet will stain the mouth red; Kaon tablets may produce a burning effect on sensitive mucosa).

Afrinol Repetabs	Drixoral tablet	Nitrospan capsule
Allerest Capsule	Ecotrin tablet	Ornade Spansule
Aminodur Duratab	E-Mycin tablet	Quinaglute Duratab
Artane Sequel	Entozyme tablet	Quinidex Extentab
ASA Enseals	Feosol tablet	Slow K tablet
Azulfadine Entab	Feosol Spansule	Sudafed SA Capsule
Bellergal-S Tablet	Ferro Grad-500 Tab	Theo-Dur tablet
Compazine Spansule	Isordil Sublingual	Ten-K
Diamox Sequel	Kaon tablet	Trental
Donnatol Extentab	Nitroglycerin tab	

From McKenry LM, Salerno E: *Mosby's pharmacology in nursing*, ed 18, St Louis, 1992, Mosby–Year Book.

Sublingual Administration

Sublingual medications are those that are placed under the tongue and allowed to dissolve. Absorption occurs across the rich supply of superficial vessels under the tongue. By far the most frequently used sublingual drugs are the nitrates and nitrites, which are used as treatment for anginal pain. Nitroglycerin is one example of a nitrate commonly administered by the sublingual route in prehospital care.

Two important points to remember when administering sublingual medications are: (1) the patient should allow the medication to dissolve completely to achieve maximum therapeutic dose, and (2) the patient should not swallow until the drug is dissolved or take oral fluids while the drug is dissolving.

Buccal Administration

Buccal tablets are manufactured so that the drug dissolves when placed and held between the cheek and gum. Like sublingual medications, buccal medications are absorbed across the oral mucosa. Also like sublingual medication, buccal medications should be allowed to dissolve entirely, and the patient should not drink any fluids while the drug is dissolving. This route is used infrequently in the prehospital setting.

Rectal Administration

Rectal administration of a drug is usually indicated for nonacute situations when the patient cannot take an oral form of the drug. An example is the patient who is vomiting. Although an antiemetic may be indicated in this situation, the oral form of the drug would probably be vomited before absorption could occur. A rectal suppository is, therefore, much more effective. Suppositories are a drug form that generally remain in solid form while at room temperature but melt when in contact with the very warm rectal

---

RECTAL ADMINISTRATION OF DIAZEPAM[3]

1. Measure the correct dose using a syringe.
2. Connect the syringe to a 10 Fr. suction catheter.
3. Lubricate the catheter.
4. Insert the catheter 3 to 5 cm into the rectum.
5. Instill the diazepam.
6. Follow with a 5 ml flush of normal saline to clear the catheter.

mucosa. Usually the drug is mixed with cocoa butter or glycerin to form the rectal suppository.

Rectal administration of drugs has not been commonplace in the prehospital setting. However, the rectal route is being used with increasing frequency for administration of diazepam in pediatric patients (see box on page 37).

Inhalation

Because the respiratory tract offers an enormous absorption surface, drugs administered via this route have both local and systemic effects. Therefore drugs administered by inhalation in the prehospital setting are usually for respiratory emergencies. Drugs administered in this manner are given in the form of a fine mist or spray. The drug is delivered into the oropharynx via a **nebulizer** or **metered-dose inhaler** while the patient is instructed to take a slow, deep breath, thereby inhaling the drug. The effect of the drug is nearly instantaneous. Techniques for administration of drugs via nebulizer or metered-dose inhaler are discussed in Chapter 7.

Endotracheal Administration

A route that is used frequently in emergencies is the endotracheal route. In instances in which there is difficulty starting an IV or there is no time for the venipuncture procedure, the endotracheal route has proven to be as effective as the IV route for some emergency medications, such as epinephrine and lidocaine.[1] Because of the capillary network of the lungs, drugs that are administered down an endotracheal tube are absorbed into the vascular system quickly.

Prior to endotracheal administration, drugs should be diluted in at least 10 ml sterile saline to facilitate absorption.[6] One word of caution: when instilling medications into an endotracheal tube, *the needle should be removed from the syringe to prevent inadvertent puncture of the tube.* A break in the integrity of an endotracheal tube can prevent adequate ventilation of an intubated patient. Also, the needle may become detached from the syringe and obstruct the tube. Some preloaded syringes do not have removable needles and in the interest of time are used as is. In such situations great care should be taken to prevent damaging the endotracheal tube with the needle.

Endotracheal administration does not negate the need to establish IV access as soon as possible. Factors that affect absorption and distribution of drugs administered endotracheally are still under investigation. There is evidence that endotracheal administration of emergency drugs is not as reliable as intravenous administration (see box on page 39).[2]

ENDOTRACHEAL DRUG ADMINISTRATION

1. Obtain order from medical control.
2. Dilute drug in 10 ml normal saline. (Many drug are diluted as packaged.)
3. Remove the needle from the syringe if possible and instill the medication into the endotracheal tube. The American Heart Association recommends passing a catheter beyond the tip of the endotracheal tube and administering the medication through the catheter.
4. If cardiopulmonary resuscitation (CPR) is being done, interrupt chest compressions briefly while the drug is instilled into the endotracheal tube.
5. Follow instillation of drug with two to three ventilations via bag-valve mask to disperse the drug.
6. Resume CPR.
7. Assess the patient's response.

Drugs that can be given endotracheally include naloxone, atropine, epinephrine, and lidocaine. Although diazepam has been given endotracheally in the past, its endotracheal use is controversial because diazepam is not water soluble and can be damaging to lung tissue.

INJECTION TECHNIQUES

As with any invasive technique, **universal precautions** should be observed for all injections (see box on page 40). Gloves should be worn for all injections and great care should be taken to prevent inadvertent needlesticks. In both the hospital and prehospital settings, needles require special handling. Needles should not be recapped but instead disposed of in an appropriate biohazard container (Figure 3-1).

Before actual techniques for injecting drugs are addressed, proper techniques for preparing injectable medications will be discussed. Many emergency drugs are supplied in preloaded syringes that are easily assembled for use (Figure 3-2). Other drugs require special preparation before they can be injected. This preparation may be as simple as withdrawing the medication from a rubber-topped vial or may require a powder to be reconstituted with a sterile fluid before it can be injected.

Syringes

A syringe is comprised of three parts: the barrel, the plunger, and the tip (Figure 3-3). The barrel is calibrated in milliliters (ml), cubic centimeters (cc), or minims (ℳ) for measuring drug volumes. The plunger fits into the

UNIVERSAL PRECAUTIONS

In an effort to protect health-care providers against bloodborne pathogens the Centers for Disease Control recommends that universal precautions be used whenever there is the potential for exposure to body fluids. Universal precautions include the use of barrier protection, such as gloves, masks, gowns, and protective eye wear. In the prehospital setting gloves are worn for all patient contact. Gowns, masks, and eyewear should be used whenever there is the potential for blood or body fluids to come in contact with one's clothing or face. In addition to protective clothing, universal precautions call for the appropriate disposal of needles and other sharps and hand washing immediately following patient contact.

The Occupational Safety and Health Administration requires that all health-care agencies provide adequate training, protective clothing, gloves, masks, eyewear and biohazard containers for health-care providers in their employ. Paramedics, whether paid or volunteer, must follow the published regulations.

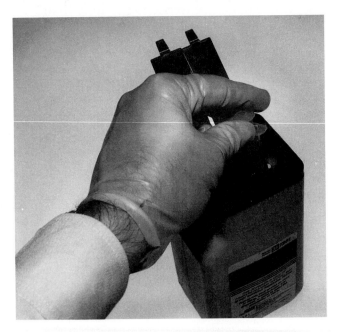

Figure 3-1 Biohazard container for needle disposal.

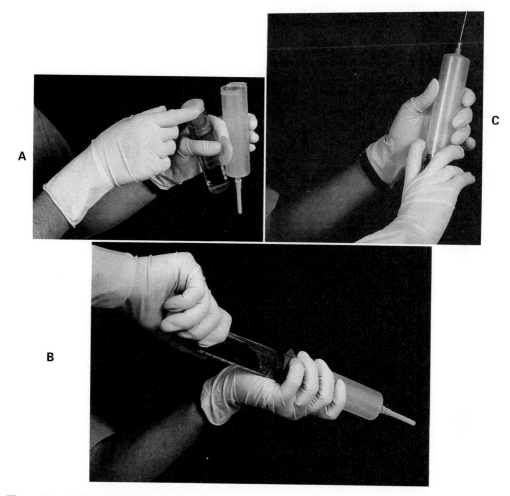

Figure 3-2   Preloaded syringes are easily assembled for use. **A,** Remove protective caps. **B,** Screw glass container (plunger) into the plastic barrel of the syringe. **C,** Push barrel in to clear air and inject drug.

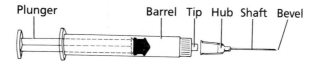

Figure 3-3   Parts of a syringe and needle. (From Perry AG, Potter PA: *Clinical Nursing Skills and Techniques*, ed 2, St Louis, Mosby–Year Book.)

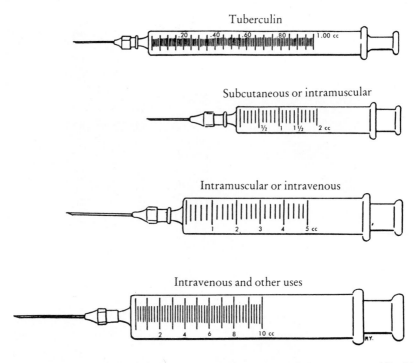

Figure 3-4 Syringes. These syringes are used to accurately measure varying amounts of liquids and liquid medications. The uppermost syringe is known as a tuberculin syringe and is graduated in 0.01 ml. It is a syringe of choice for administration of very small amounts. The 2 ml syringe is the one commonly used to give a drug subcutaneously or intramuscularly. It is graduated in 0.1 ml. The larger syringes are used when a larger volume of drug is to be administered intramuscularly or intravenously, for withdrawing blood for laboratory testing, or for obtaining urine specimens from urinary catheters (20-ml syringes may be preferred for the last two uses). These syringes and needles are not drawn to scale (e.g., the tuberculin syringe is much thinner and shorter than the others). (From McKenry LM, Salerno E: *Mosby's Pharmacology in Nursing*, ed 18, St Louis, 1992, Mosby–Year Book.)

barrel and is moved back and forth to draw up and inject medications. The tip is the part of the syringe to which the needle is attached. Syringes are available in a variety of sizes (Figure 3-4).

Needles

A needle has three parts: the hub, the shaft, and the beveled tip (Figure 3-3). The needle gauge refers to the diameter of the hole through the needle (commonly referred to as the bore). The larger the gauge number, the smaller the bore. For example, an 18-gauge needle has a larger diameter than a 20-gauge needle. The needle gauge is selected on the basis of the viscosity of the fluid to be injected. The length of the shaft of the needle is selected on the basis of the depth of penetration desired.

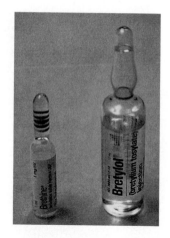

Figure 3-5   Ampules.

Withdrawing Medication from Glass Ampules

Some emergency drugs are supplied in small glass ampules that are intended for single-dose use only (Figure 3-5). The ampules are designed so that they can easily be broken for withdrawal of the medication.

Frequently the cap of the ampule traps a portion of the drug; however, the drug can easily be freed from the cap by spinning the ampule between the hands. Paramedics should hold the ampule with an alcohol wipe or sterile gauze when breaking the top to prevent cuts from broken shards of glass. A syringe with a filter needle should be used when drawing medications out of a glass ampule, as small glass particles may fall into the ampule when the top is broken off. Filter needles are used routinely in the hospital setting but are not always available to paramedics in the field.

Although withdrawing medication from the ampule may seem clumsy at first, the student will become very comfortable with practice. As always, asepsis is of the utmost importance. Care should be taken not to contaminate the needle or the medication when withdrawing the medication from the ampule (Figure 3-6).

Withdrawing Drugs from Rubber-Topped Vials

Injectable medications are commonly supplied in rubber-topped vials (Figure 3-7). The vials may be designed for either single-dose or multiple-dose use.

A needle and syringe are used to withdraw drugs from rubber-topped vials. A volume of air equivalent in volume to the amount of medication to be withdrawn must first be injected into the vial to prevent the formation of

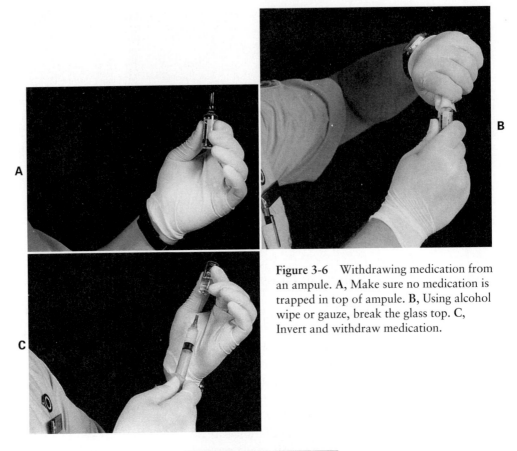

Figure 3-6   Withdrawing medication from an ampule. **A,** Make sure no medication is trapped in top of ampule. **B,** Using alcohol wipe or gauze, break the glass top. **C,** Invert and withdraw medication.

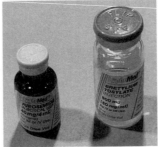

Figure 3-7   Vials.

a vacuum. For example, to withdraw 10 ml from a vial, 10 ml of air should first be injected. Then with the needle still inserted in the vial, the vial is turned upside down and 10 ml of fluid is withdrawn. When a larger volume medication is to be withdrawn (e.g., 30 ml), it is often necessary to repeat the process several times. Figure 3-8 depicts use of a rubber-topped vial.

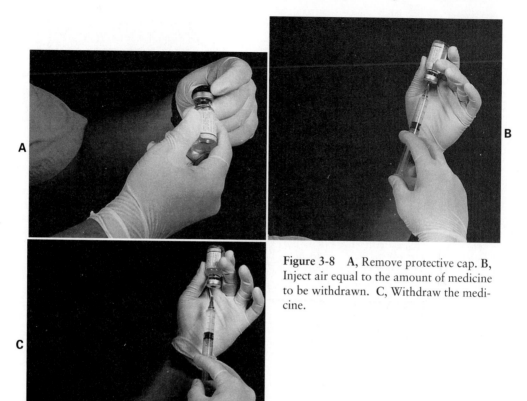

Figure 3-8 **A,** Remove protective cap. **B,** Inject air equal to the amount of medicine to be withdrawn. **C,** Withdraw the medicine.

Intradermal Injection

An infrequently used technique in emergency medicine, intradermal injection is most often used in allergy testing and for administration of local anesthetics. In some EMS systems in which paramedics insert central venous lines, local anesthetics may be injected intradermally to anesthetize the insertion site. The injection is made just under the outer layer of skin (Figure 3-9), using a small-bore needle (25- to 27-gauge) and a small-volume syringe. Generally, no more than 1 ml should be injected intradermally.

Procedure
1. Explain procedure to the patient.
2. Wash hands; don gloves.
3. Select the appropriate sized needle and syringe (Table 3-3). Withdraw the medication from the vial or ampule.

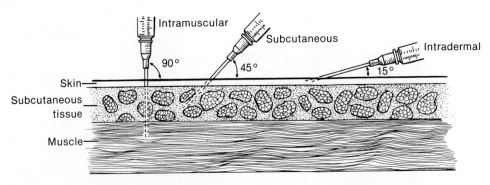

Figure 3-9 Comparison of angles of insertion for intramuscular (90 degrees), subcutaneous (45 degrees), and intradermal (15 degrees) injections. (From Perry AG, Potter PA: *Clinical Nursing Skills and Techniques*, ed 2, St Louis, 1990, Mosby–Year Book.)

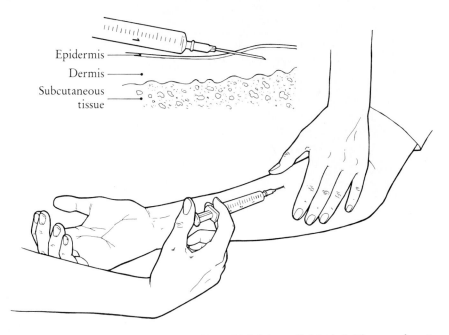

Figure 3-10 Intradermal injection. (From McKenry LM, Salerno E: *Mosby's Pharmacology in Nursing*, ed 18, St Louis, 1992, Mosby–Year Book.)

4. Cleanse the chosen insertion site with alcohol. The most frequently used site for intradermal injection is the medial aspect of the anterior forearm. Alcohol should be allowed to dry completely before proceeding.
5. Holding the skin taut with one hand, insert the needle at a 10- to 15-degree angle (Figure 3-10). The prescribed amount is then gently injected to form a wheal, which is a raised area resembling a mosquito

Table 3-3 Suggested Injection Guides

ROUTE	COMMON AREAS	REGION	VOLUME INJECTED (ml)			EXAMPLES OF MEDICATIONS BY THIS ROUTE
			NEEDLE SIZES	AVERAGE	RANGE	
Intradermal (intracutaneous)	Skin (corium)	Inner aspect of mid forearm or scapula	26 or 27 gauge × $\frac{3}{8}$ in	0.1	0.001 to 1.0	Tuberculin, allergens, local anesthetics
Subcutaneous	Beneath the skin	Lateral upper arm; thighs; abdominal fat pads except the 1-in area around umbilicus and tissue over bone; upper back; upper hips	25 to 27 gauge × $\frac{1}{2}$ to $\frac{5}{8}$ in	0.5	0.5 to 1.5	Epinephrine (non-oily), insulin, some narcotics, tetanus toxoid, vaccines, vitamin B_{12}, heparin
Intramuscular	Gluteus medius	Dorsogluteal	20 to 23 gauge × $1\frac{1}{2}$ to 3 in	2 to 4	1 to 5	Most intramuscular and Z-track injections
	Gluteus minimus	Ventrogluteal	20 to 23 gauge × $1\frac{1}{2}$ to 3 in	1 to 4	1 to 5	All intramuscular medications
	Vastus lateralis	Anterolateral midthigh	22 to 25 gauge × $\frac{5}{8}$ to 1 in	1 to 4	1 to 5	Almost all intramuscular medications
	Deltoid	Upper arm below shoulder	23 to 25 gauge × $\frac{5}{8}$ to 1 in	0.5	0.5 to 2	Vaccines, absorbed tetanus toxoid, most narcotics, epinephrine, sedatives, vitamin B_{12}, lidocaine
Intravenous bolus	Cephalic and basilic veins	Dorsum of hand and forearm; antecubital fossa	18 to 23 gauge × 1 to $1\frac{1}{2}$ in	1 to 10	0.5 to 50 (or more by continuous infusion)	Antibiotics, vitamins, fluids and electrolytes, antineoplastics, vasopressors, corticosteroids, aminophylline, and blood products

From McKenry LM, Salerno E: *Pharmacology in nursing*, ed 18, St Louis, 1992, Mosby–Year Book.

bite. If a wheal does not form or if the site bleeds, the injection was probably given too deeply. Depending on the reason for the injection, it may need to be repeated.

Subcutaneous Injection

Subcutaneous injection is commonly used in emergency medicine. The medication is injected into the loose connective tissue between the dermis and muscle layer (see Figure 3-9). Epinephrine, terbutaline, and insulin are examples of drugs that can be administered subcutaneously. Generally, the volume injected should be no more than 1.5 ml.

Procedure
1. Explain procedure to the patient.
2. Wash hands; don gloves.
3. Select the appropriate sized needle and syringe (see Table 3-3).
4. Select the appropriate injection site (Figure 3-11).
5. Cleanse the site thoroughly with alcohol, and allow it to dry before proceeding. In emergency situations it is acceptable to wipe the site dry with a sterile gauze pad or sponge (Figure 3-12).

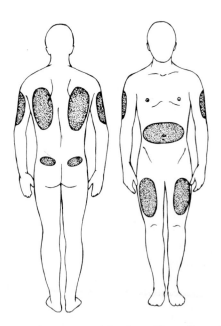

Figure 3-11 Common sites for subcutaneous injections. (From Perry AG, Potter PA: *Clinical Nursing Skills and Techniques*, ed 2, St Louis, 1990, Mosby–Year Book.)

6. Pinch the skin up slightly between the thumb and other fingers.
7. Insert the needle using a quick, dartlike motion, using the appropriate angle (Figure 3-13). When using a ⅝-inch needle, a 45-degree angle should be used with most adults. In very obese patients, the angle of insertion should be increased to 60 degrees. Conversely, in

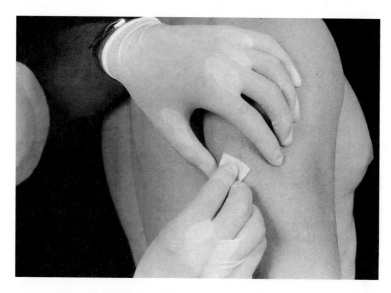

Figure 3-12   Cleanse the injection site.

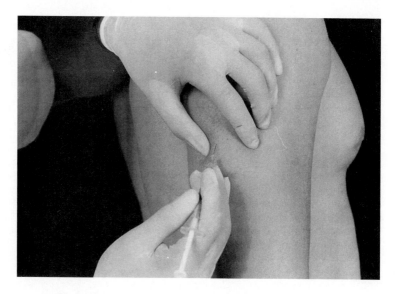

Figure 3-13   Insert needle with a quick, dart-like motion.

very thin or emaciated patients, the angle of injection should be reduced to 30 degrees. With a ½-inch needle, the angle of insertion is 90 degrees. Before injecting, slightly aspirate to check for blood to ensure that the drug will not be injected directly into a blood vessel. Should blood be drawn into the syringe, the needle should be withdrawn. The medication should be discarded and another dose prepared.

8. Gently inject the medication (Figure 3-14).
9. Remove the needle
10. Discard the needle in an appropriate container.
11. Massage the injection site to reduce discomfort and disperse medication.

Intramuscular Injection

The IM injection route allows medication to be inserted directly into the muscle (Figure 3-9). It has several advantages over the subcutaneous route: larger amounts of fluid can be injected (up to 5 ml), absorption is faster, and drugs that are irritating to the tissues are better tolerated when given IM. For volumes larger than 3 ml to 5 ml, more than one injection site can be used.

To inject into a muscle a longer needle must be used (see Table 3-3). Because of the depth of IM injection, special care must be taken to avoid damaging nerves. Accidental injection of a nerve can result in permanent

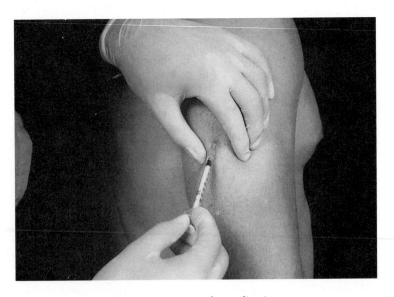

Figure 3-14   Inject the medication.

disability for the patient. For this reason it is necessary to learn to map the appropriate injection sites by use of landmarks. Sites used for IM injection include the arm (deltoid), the thigh (rectus femoris or vastus lateralis), and the hip (dorsogluteal or ventrogluteal).

The deltoid muscle site, located in the lateral aspect of the upper arm, is an easily accessible site (Figure 3-15). It is better perfused than other sites for IM injection, making it a good site for emergency drugs. It does, however, have several disadvantages. It can only accommodate small amounts of

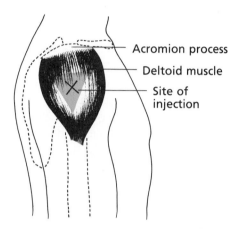

Figure 3-15 Site of intramuscular injection into deltoid muscle. (From Perry AG, Potter PA: *Clinical Nursing Skills and Techniques*, ed 2, St Louis, 1990, Mosby–Year Book.)

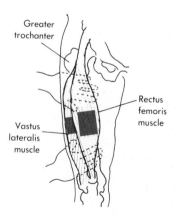

Figure 3-16 To define the vastus lateralis muscle injection site and the rectus femoris muscle site, place one hand below the patient's greater trochanter and one hand above the knee. The space between the two hands defines the middle third of the underlying muscle. The rectus femoris is on the anterior thigh; the vastus lateralis is on the lateral thigh. (From Clark JB, Queener SF, Karb VB: *Pharmacological Basis of Nursing Practice*, ed 3, St Louis, 1990, Mosby–Year Book.)

fluid (1 ml in women and children and up to 2 ml in well-developed males). Also, it is in close proximity to the radial nerve.

The vastus lateralis and rectus femoris sites are adjacent muscles in the thigh (Figure 3-16). To find these sites the paramedic should place one hand on the patient's upper thigh and one hand on the lower thigh. The area between the two hands is the appropriate area for injection. The rectus femoris is on the anterior surface at the midline (Figure 3-17), whereas the vastus lateralis is lateral to the midline (Figure 3-18). Up to 3 ml can be injected in the average adult and up to 5 ml can be injected in a well-developed muscle at these sites. The vastus lateralis and rectus femoris are the preferred sites for IM injections in infants.

The ventrogluteal site is best accessed by having the patient lie supine. To locate the site place the palm of the hand on the greater trochanter (Figure 3-19). Form a "V" with the index and middle fingers pointing toward the anterior iliac spine and the iliac crest. The injection should be made within the V. The ventrogluteal site is particularly useful in the prehospital setting, as it can accommodate large volumes of medication and does not require that the patient be moved from a supine position. In the well-developed adult this site can accommodate up to 5 ml of fluid. This site can also be used in children.

The dorsogluteal site is identified by locating the greater trochanter and the posterior superior iliac spine. An imaginary line is drawn between the two, and the injection is made in the area between the imaginary line and the curve of the iliac crest (Figure 3-20). To best identify the landmarks used for

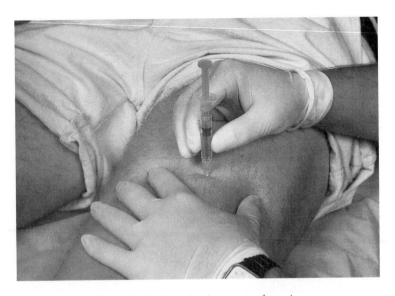

Figure 3-17   Injection into rectus femoris.

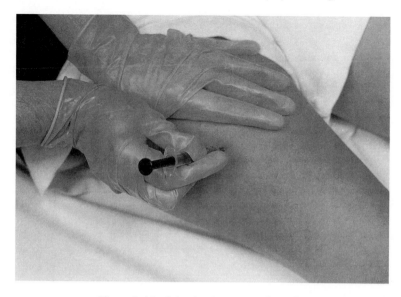

Figure 3-18   Injection into vastus lateralis.

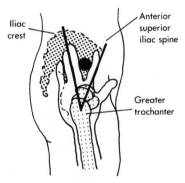

Figure 3-19   To locate the ventrogluteal muscle injection site, place the palm of one hand on the greater trochanter of the femur. Make a "V" with the fingers of that hand, with one side running from the greater trochanter to the anterosuperior iliac spine and the other side running from the greater trochanter to the iliac crest. (From Clark JB, Queener SF, Karb VB: *Pharmacological Basis of Nursing Practice*, ed 3, St Louis, 1990, Mosby–Year Book.)

locating this site it is advisable to have the patient in a prone position. As an alternative, a side-lying position is sufficient. Accuracy in identifying the dorsogluteal site is particularly important because of the proximity of the gluteal artery and the sciatic nerve. The dorsogluteal site is not recommended for infants. Figure 3-21 illustrates administration of a dorsogluteal injection.

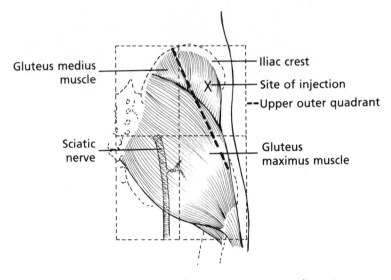

Figure 3-20   Imaginary diagonal line extending from posterior superior iliac spine to greater trochanter is landmark for selecting dorsogluteal injection site. Alternatively, buttocks may be divided into quadrants for selecting dorsogluteal injection site. (From Perry AG, Potter PA: *Clinical Nursing Skills and Techniques*, ed 2, St Louis, 1990, Mosby–Year Book.)

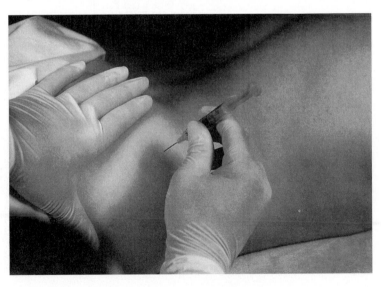

Figure 3-21   Dorsogluteal injection.

Procedure

1. Explain procedure to the patient.
2. Wash hands; don gloves.
3. Select the appropriate sized needle and syringe (see Table 3-3).
4. Select the appropriate injection site. Factors to be considered in site selection include:
   - ability of the patient to cooperate
   - amount of drug to be given
   - type of drug to be given (very irritating drugs should be given in the large gluteal muscles).
5. Cleanse the site thoroughly with alcohol, and allow it to dry before proceeding (Figure 3-22). In emergency situations it is acceptable to wipe the site dry with a sterile gauze pad.
6. Insert the needle using a quick, dartlike motion (Figure 3-23). Aspirate before injecting to check for blood return (Figure 3-24). Inject the drug gently. IM injections should be made at a 90-degree angle, perpendicular to the surface of the skin (Figure 3-25).
7. Remove the needle.
8. Discard the needle in an appropriate container.
9. Massage the site to reduce discomfort and disperse medication.

A technique that is especially useful for IM injection of drugs that are irritating to the tissues and thus painful to the patient is the **Z**-track tech-

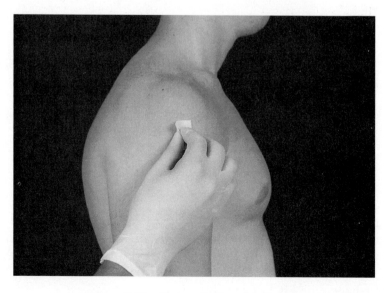

Figure 3-22 Cleanse the site with alcohol.

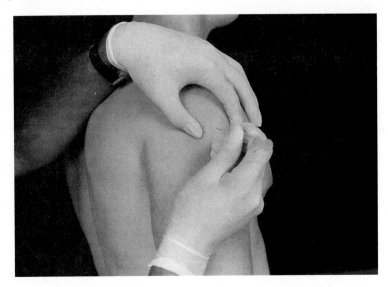

Figure 3-23 Using a dart-like motion, inject the site.

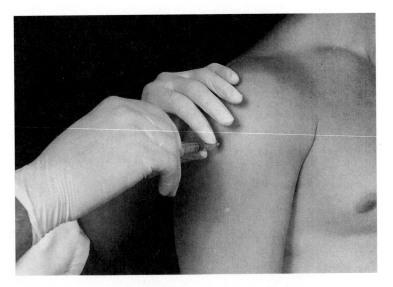

Figure 3-24 Aspirate.

nique (Figure 3-26). Although this technique can be used with any IM injection, it is most commonly used with the dorsogluteal site. This technique prevents medication from leaking back into the SC tissue once it is injected. An example of a drug that should be given using the Z-track technique is hydroxyzine HCl (Vistaril).

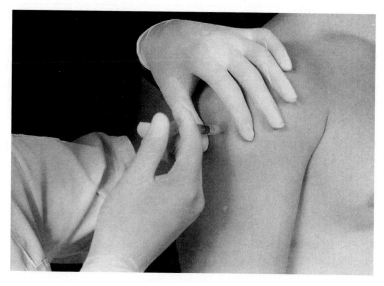

Figure 3-25   Inject the drug slowly.

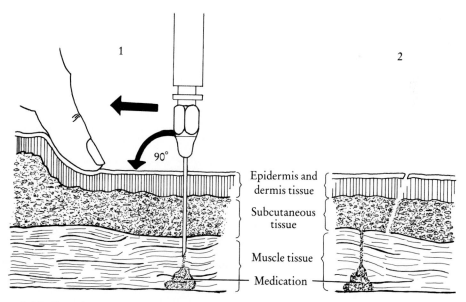

Figure 3-26 Z-track intramuscular injection method, which is useful for administration of medication known to cause pain or permanent staining of superficial tissues. 1, The skin is stretched to one side and medication injected as usual, perpendicular to the skin surface; 2, needle is then removed and the skin allowed to return to resting position, sealing off the deposited medication from the track made by the needle. The site is not massaged in this method. (From McKenry LM, Salerno E: *Mosby's Pharmacology in Nursing*, ed 18, St Louis, 1992, Mosby–Year Book.)

INTRAVENOUS ADMINISTRATION OF DRUGS

IV therapy refers to the administration of fluids and/or drugs directly into venous circulation. IV therapy is an important aspect of the management of medical and traumatic emergencies. There are three reasons for initiating IV therapy: (1) to replace fluid; (2) to establish venous access for the administration of medications; and (3) to obtain blood samples. The IV route is the most commonly used route for drug administration in the prehospital and emergency settings. Administering a drug intravenously places the medication directly into the bloodstream. The onset of action is, therefore, more rapid than with all other parenteral routes. IV administration also permits large volumes to be given and is generally more comfortable for the patient than IM or SC injections. On the other hand, time and skill are required to perform a venipuncture and establish an IV line (commonly referred to as an IV).

Venipuncture refers to the technique of inserting a needle or catheter through the skin and into a vein for the purpose of withdrawing a blood specimen or administering drugs and/or fluid. The remainder of this chapter discusses the technique of venipuncture and the administration of IV medications. IV fluid therapy is discussed in Chapter 5.

Establishing an IV

Equipment. A list of equipment required for initiating an IV is presented in the box below.

EQUIPMENT FOR INITIATING AN INTRAVENOUS INFUSION

1. Gloves
2. IV fluid
3. Solution set
4. IV catheter or needle
5. Prep pads (betadine or alcohol)
6. Tourniquet
7. Antibacterial ointment
8. Tape
9. Dressing

KEY TERM

Venipuncture—insertion of a needle or catheter through the skin into a vein for the purpose of administering fluid or drugs or for obtaining a blood specimen.

Gloves should be worn throughout the IV procedure to prevent exposure to blood. The Centers for Disease Control recommends that universal blood and body fluid precautions be used in all situations in which there is a risk of exposure to blood or other body fluids.

There are a variety of administration sets available today, all of which are similar in principle (Figures 3-27*A* and 3-27*B*). An administration set consists of (1) a drip chamber, which is spiked at the proximal end for insertion into the fluid bag or bottle; (2) plastic tubing, whose distal end is designed to insert directly into the IV needle or catheter; (3) a roller clamp that permits regulation of the rate of administration; and (4) an injection port.

The number of drops required to deliver 1 ml of solution is referred to as the drop factor. The *micro* or *mini* drip has a ratio of 60 drops per ml (Figure 3-28). The mini drip solution set is used when small volumes of fluid or medication are to be administered. The *standard* or *macro* drip provides a drop factor of 10, 15, or 20 drops per ml (Figure 3-29). The specific drop factor is indicated on the package by the manufacturer. The macro drip is selected when large volumes of fluid need to be given.

Some administration sets are equipped with a volume control chamber that permits only a specified amount of fluid to be administered (Figure 3-30). It is connected to the required fluid, and the desired amount is run into the fluid chamber. A clamp between the fluid source and the fluid chamber is then closed, preventing additional fluid from entering the chamber. The volume control chamber is used when it is important to carefully regulate the volume of fluid being given, such as fluid administration for infants and children or for those patients with severe fluid restrictions.

There is also a specialized tubing for the administration of whole blood and blood products. This tubing is referred to as a blood solution set or y-

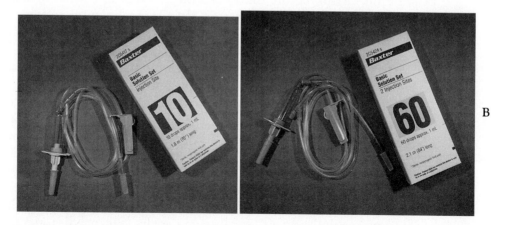

Figure 3-27 Administration sets. **A,** Administration set with standard or macrodrip. **B,** Administration set with microdrip.

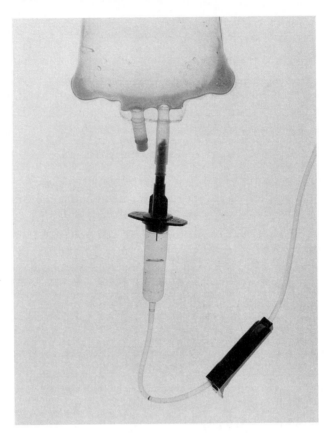

Figure 3-28   Microdrip or minidrip chamber (60 gtt/ml).

tubing (Figure 3-31). The y-tubing allows normal saline to be infused when priming the tubing before blood is administered and when flushing the tubing following blood administration. In the prehospital setting, a y-tubing can be used for fluid resuscitation or in anticipation of blood administration upon arrival at the hospital.

There are two types of IV catheters or needles commonly used today. They are available in a variety of lengths and gauges:

1. Over-the-needle catheters—The majority of IVs in the emergency setting are started with over-the-needle catheters (Figures 3-32*A* and 3-32*B*). These consist of a flexible catheter over a stainless steel hollow needle.

2. Scalp vein or butterfly—The scalp vein needle or butterfly needle is a stainless steel hollow needle that is inserted and taped in place (Figure 3-33). The stainless steel needles are generally used in non-emergent situations when the duration of IV therapy is short. In the prehospital setting, small-gauge scalp vein needles are occasionally used for children or elderly adults.

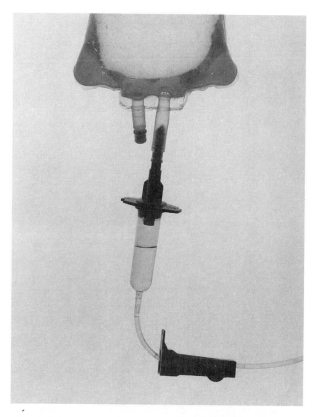

Figure 3-29   Standard or macrodrip chamber (10 gtt/ml).

The general rule to follow when selecting a catheter is to choose the smallest bore that will accomplish the purpose for which the IV is being started. The larger the needle diameter, the greater the flow rate. Catheters used for peripheral IVs are generally 1½ to 2 inches in length. Large-bore catheters (14- to 18- gauge) should be selected for patients in shock, cardiac arrest, or other life-threatening emergencies in which rapid fluid replacement is required. Also, for those patients who may require blood, an 18-gauge or larger catheter should be used. In less serious emergencies when administering IV medications is anticipated, an 18-gauge catheter is probably adequate. It is important to note that damage to the vein and other complications of IV therapy are often related to the size of the catheter being used. The larger the gauge, the more likely it is that complications will occur.

The availability of veins in a particular patient can also influence catheter selection. Paramedics must make a clinical judgment regarding the catheter size when assessing the patient's veins. For example, some elderly patients' veins cannot accommodate a large-bore catheter. Attempts to place too large a catheter can result in unsuccessful **cannulation** and lost time. In

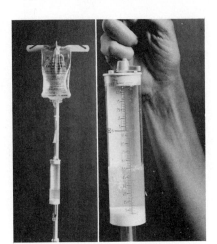

Figure 3-30 Volume control chamber. (From Perry AG, Potter PA: *Clinical Nursing Skills and Techniques*, ed 2, St Louis, 1990, Mosby–Year Book.)

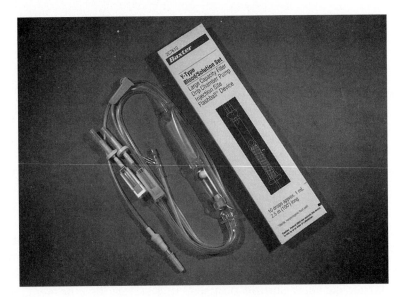

Figure 3-31 Blood solution set.

such situations it would be best to use a smaller catheter, such as a 20-gauge. In children, small-gauge catheters (21- to 24-gauge) or butterfly needles are used depending on the age and size of the child.

Selecting a vein. The veins used most frequently for IV therapy are the veins of the arms and hands. These include the metacarpal veins, dorsal vein network, basilic vein, and cephalic vein (Figures 3-34A and 3-34B). In young children and infants the veins most commonly used are those on the

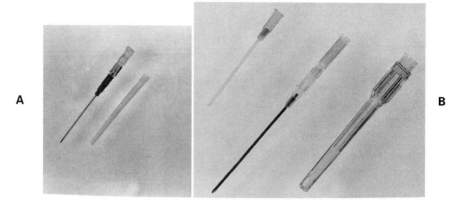

Figure 3-32 **A,** Over-the-needle catheter. **B,** Over-the-needle catheter with catheter removed.

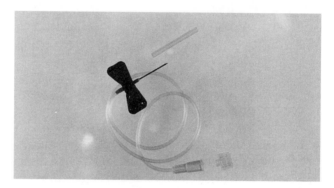

Figure 3-33 Butterfly needle.

dorsal aspect of the hand, the dorsum of the foot, and the temporal region of the scalp (Figure 3-35). The following variables should be considered when selecting a vein:

- The veins of the hand are smaller than those of the forearm and antecubital area. If the patient's condition dictates the need for a large-bore catheter, the larger veins of the forearm and antecubital area should be used.
- **Antecubital veins** should be used for patients in severe shock or cardiac arrest. These veins are usually large and more easily cannulated. In addition, circulation to distal extremities is markedly reduced in such low perfusion states. Therefore medications given in an antecubital vein reach circulation faster than those given in the hand or forearm. IV infusions started in the antecubital area are generally less comfortable for the patient as a result of the necessity of keeping the extremity immobilized.

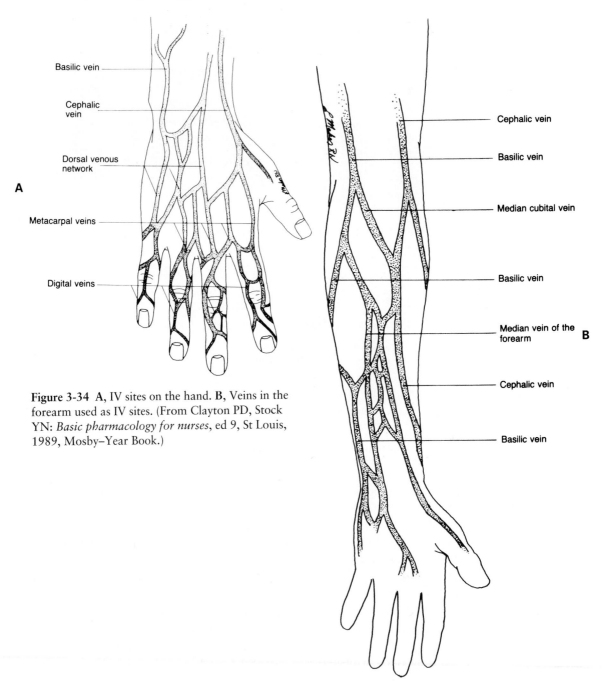

Figure 3-34 A, IV sites on the hand. **B,** Veins in the forearm used as IV sites. (From Clayton PD, Stock YN: *Basic pharmacology for nurses,* ed 9, St Louis, 1989, Mosby–Year Book.)

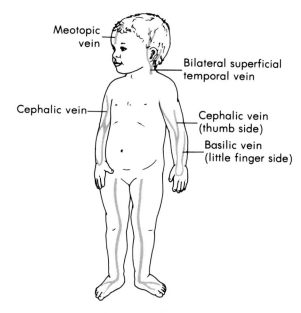

Figure 3-35 Veins in infants and children used as IV sites. (From Clayton PD, Stock YN: *Basic pharmacology for Nurses*, ed 9, St Louis, 1989, Mosby–Year Book.)

- In less urgent situations when prolonged IV therapy is a possibility, it is in the best interest of the patient to begin with the most distal vein of adequate size (usually the hand). Subsequent lines can then be placed above (proximal to) the previous site.
- The veins of the lower extremities should be used as a last resort in adults because use of these veins places the patient at increased risk for thrombus formation.
- The dorsal aspect of the hand should be avoided in the elderly because they frequently have very fragile skin and veins in this area.
- Veins over bony prominences or joints should be avoided because of the potential for the catheter or needle becoming dislodged and increased discomfort for the patient when these sites are used.
- If possible, the patient's nondominant hand should be used, freeing the dominant hand.
- When veins of the hands or arm cannot be cannulated, the external jugular vein can provide a valuable alternative site for IV therapy. The external jugular vein is a relatively large vein located in the neck below the ear and behind the angle of the mandible (Figure 3-36), which is readily visible in most adults. Because infants and children have shorter necks, the external jugular vein is more difficult to cannulate and is therefore used less frequently in pediatric patients. A disadvantage in using the external jugular vein is that the catheter and

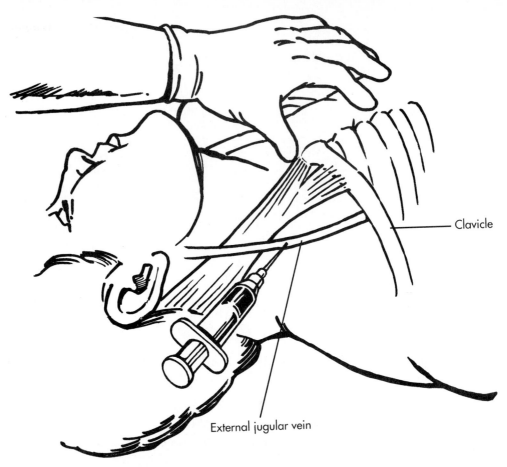

Figure 3-36 Anatomy of external jugular vein.

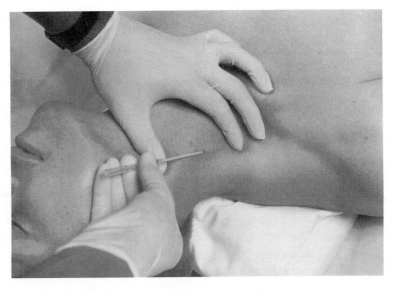

Figure 3-37 Approach to external jugular vein.

tubing are difficult to secure and can be displaced with movement of the patient's head, as occurs with endotracheal intubation or cardiopulmonary resuscitation (CPR). The box below describes the procedure for cannulating the external jugular. Figure 3-37 shows the approach to the external jugular vein.

Preparing the fluid. Fluid for IV administration is available in plastic bags and plastic or glass bottles. Plastic bags are used far more frequently than bottles.

1. Maintain aseptic technique throughout the entire procedure.
2. Check the solution. Read the label to ensure that the correct fluid is being administered, and check the expiration date (Figure 3-38). The solution should be inspected for clarity, and the bag should be checked for leaks.
3. Move the solution set from the box, maintaining sterility at both ends.
4. Place the roller clamp 1 to 2 inches below the drip chamber (Figure 3-39) and clamp the tubing.
5. Remove the protective covers from the bag and the tubing insertion spike, being careful to maintain the sterility of both (Figure 3-40).
6. Insert the spike into the bag (Figure 3-41).
7. Holding the fluid upright, squeeze the drip chamber and release to fill the drip chamber (Figure 3-42). The drip chamber should be filled about half way.
8. Remove the protective cover at the opposite end of the tubing and open the clamp to fill the tubing with fluid (Figure 3-43). All air should be cleared from the tubing.
9. Close the clamp and replace the protective cover.

PROCEDURE FOR CANNULATING THE EXTERNAL JUGULAR VEIN

1. Explain procedure to the patient.
2. Wash hands; don gloves.
3. Place the patient in a supine, head-down position (to fill the vein).
4. Turn the patient's head to the opposite side. (If the mechanism of injury suggests C-spine precautions, the external jugular site should be used only if necessary and cervical spine alignment should be maintained throughout the procedure.)
5. Cleanse the site with an antibacterial solution.
6. Apply light pressure over the vein with one finger just above the clavicle to stabilize and help fill the vein.
7. Insert the over-the-needle catheter* midway between the angle of the jaw and the midclavicular line.
8. Connect fluid as with any other IV.

---

* A large-bore catheter should be used, preferably 14- to 16-gauge.

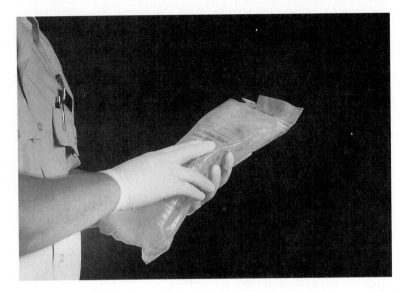

Figure 3-38   Label should be read to check expiration date and the type of fluid.

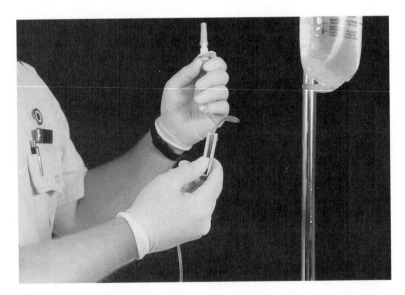

Figure 3-39   Place the roller clamp 1 to 2 inches below the drip chamber.

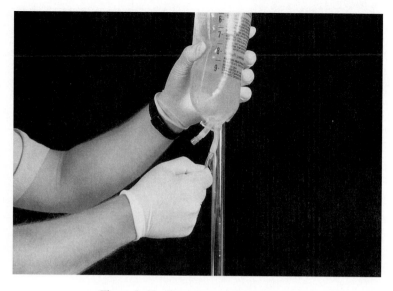

Figure 3-40 Remove protective covers.

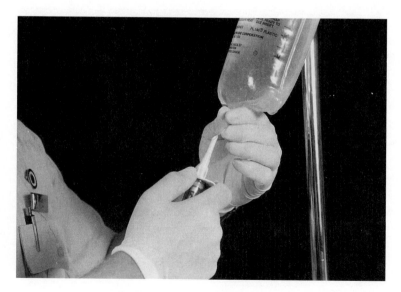

Figure 3-41 Insert spike into bag.

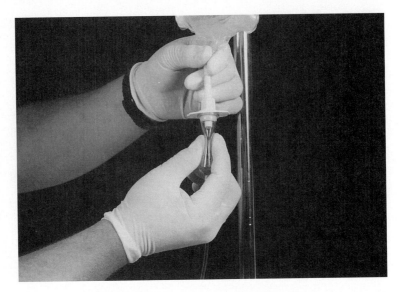

Figure 3-42   Squeeze drip chamber to fill.

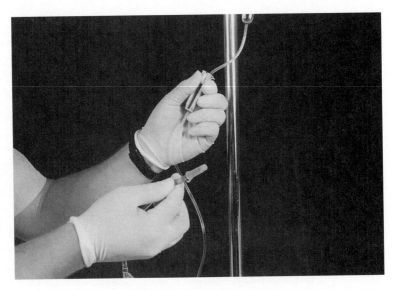

Figure 3-43   Clear air from tubing.

Performing the venipuncture

1. Explain the procedure to the patient.
2. Wash hands; don gloves.
3. Assemble the equipment.
4. Apply the tourniquet 6 to 8 inches above the intended insertion site (Figure 3-44). The tourniquet should not obstruct arterial flow. Check distal pulse.
5. Select a well-dilated vein.
6. Clean the insertion site with an antibacterial solution (Figure 3-45). Although the antibacterial solution used is determined by agency protocol, commonly used solutions are betadine or alcohol. If alcohol is used, the site should be scrubbed for 3 minutes.
7. Holding the needle at a 30-degree angle, with the bevel up, penetrate the skin approximately 1 inch below the intended entry site into the vein (Figure 3-46).
8. Once the skin has been penetrated, reduce the angle to 15 degrees and slowly advance the needle into the vein.
9. When the vein is penetrated, a blood return, or flashback, should be visible in the tubing of the butterfly or the hub of the needle in the angiocath.
10. When the blood return is observed, the butterfly needle should be advanced the entire length of the needle. With the angiocath, the needle and catheter should be advanced approximately 1/4 inch once the blood return is observed. The catheter should then be advanced its entire length while holding the needle stationary (Figure 3-47). The needle should be removed and the catheter left in place (Figure 3-48). Care should be taken in handling the needle until it can be appropriately discarded.
11. While stabilizing the catheter or needle with one hand, quickly release the tourniquet (Figure 3-49) and connect the tubing (Figure 3-50). One of the most common reasons why an IV does not run is that the tourniquet is not removed at this point.
12. Open the clamp slowly and observe for a rapid flow rate to ensure patency. Reduce to a slow rate (10 to 20 gtts/min).
13. Place antiseptic ointment at the insertion site.
14. Tape the catheter or needle in place (Figure 3-51).
15. Apply a sterile dressing.
16. The time, date, needle size, and the paramedic's initials should be written on the outside of the dressing.
17. Adjust the rate as prescribed.

Text continued on page 76.

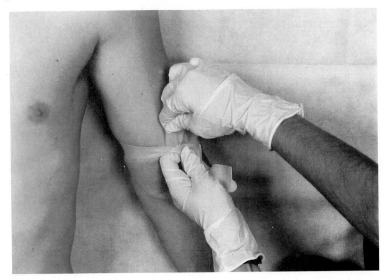

Figure 3-44   Apply tourniquet 6 to 8 inches above the insertion site.

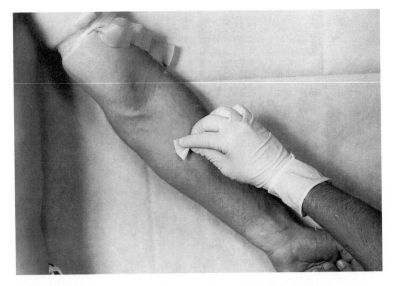

Figure 3-45   Cleanse the insertion site.

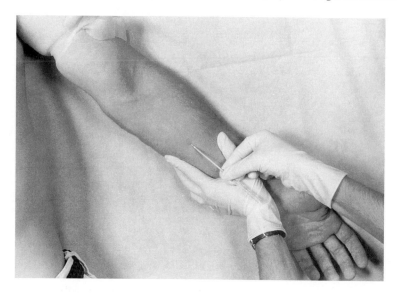

Figure 3-46   Enter skin at a 30-degree angle with bevel up.

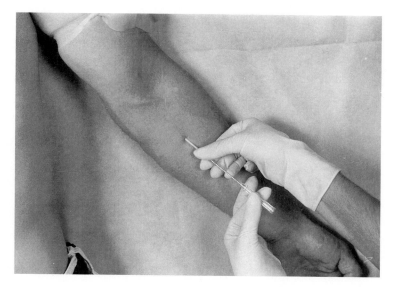

Figure 3-47   Advance the catheter.

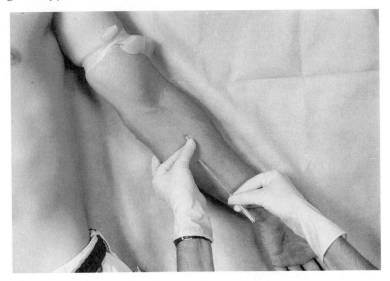

Figure 3-48   Remove the needle.

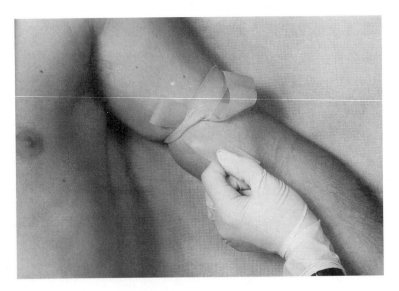

Figure 3-49   Release the tourniquet.

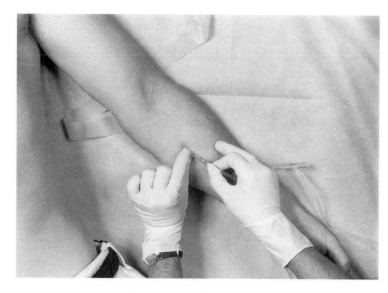

Figure 3-50   Connect the tubing.

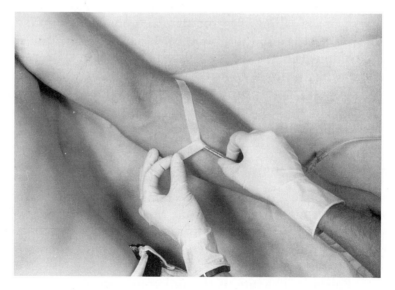

Figure 3-51   Tape the catheter in place.

18. Discard supplies. Needles and any other supplies contaminated with blood should be discarded in an appropriate biohazard container. *Needles should not be recapped.*

Regulating flow rates. Once the IV line is established, paramedics are responsible for regulating the rate of infusion as prescribed by the physician. In severe cases of shock, fluids are infused at a very rapid rate (see Chapter 5 for a discussion of rapid infusions). The physician may order that the IV be run *wide open,* which means the clamp is opened completely and the fluid is allowed to infuse as quickly as possible. One liter of fluid can be infused in as little as 5 minutes with a large-bore catheter and tubing in a large vein. When the infusion is intended to provide venous access only (rather than replace fluid), the IV is referred to as a *keep open.* For example, the order may be to start 500 ml D_5W TKO (to keep open). A keep-open rate is a rate just adequate enough to keep the IV infusing, generally less than 50 ml per hour.

In the hospital setting infusion pumps and IV controllers are frequently used to regulate and monitor infusion rates (see box on page 77). Although these devices are used less frequently in the field, they are available in some services. When controllers or infusion pumps are not used, paramedics must manually control the infusion rate by adjusting the roller clamp on the IV tubing. The infusion rate is assessed by counting the number of drops falling into the drip chamber per minute. Drops are counted for 15 seconds and multiplied by 4. The infusion rate should be monitored continuously because administering too much or too little fluid can be deleterious to the patient. Changes in the patient's position can significantly change the infusion rate. This is particularly true in a moving ambulance. The middle box on page 77 provides tips on trouble-shooting IVs that do not infuse.

Complications of Intravenous Therapy

There are a number of potential complications associated with IV therapy. Many of the complications do not occur until several hours after the initiation of IV therapy and are therefore not usually seen by paramedics. However, infiltration and fluid overload can occur rapidly and should be of concern to paramedics.

Phlebitis. Phlebitis is the inflammation of a vein caused by mechanical irritation from a needle or catheter, or by chemical irritation from certain medications. Phlebitis does not usually occur in the first hours of IV therapy, so it is usually not observed until the patient has been admitted to the hospital. Phlebitis is characterized by pain, redness, and swelling at the insertion site and along the vein tract. Phlebitis can predispose the patient to clot formation. The inflammation associated with clot formation is referred to as

thrombophlebitis. Should the clot become dislodged, the resulting **thromboembolism** can cause obstruction of pulmonary blood flow (pulmonary embolism), coronary blood flow (coronary embolism), or cerebral blood flow (cerebral embolism). Thrombophlebitis is characterized by localized heat, redness, swelling, and hardness of the vein.

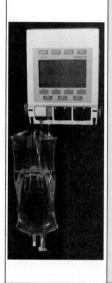

INFUSION CONTROLLERS AND PUMPS

Infusion controllers and infusion pumps provide for more accurate regulation of IV flow rates than is possible to achieve with a simple roller clamp. These are small, battery-powered, boxlike devices that are attached to an IV pole or mounted to the wall of the ambulance or helicopter. Infusion controllers work simply by using gravity and are less accurate than infusion pumps.

There are two types of infusion pumps: nonvolumetric and volumetric. Nonvolumetric pumps measure fluid volume by drop rate. Volumetric pumps infuse solutions very precisely in milliliters per hour. Volumetric pumps are typically used for the administration of potent drugs by continuous infusion, such as dopamine, isoproterenol, streptokinase, and nitroprusside.

There are a variety of controllers and pumps available commercially. Many interhospital transfers require the use of controllers and pumps, but the degree to which they are used in EMS varies.

TROUBLESHOOTING IV LINES

In the event that an IV will not infuse, the following steps should be taken:

1. Ensure that the tourniquet has been removed.
2. Check the line for kinks or obstruction caused by the patient or nearby equipment.
3. Check to see that the roller clamp and line clamps are open.
4. Raise the height of the IV infusion bag.
5. Gently manipulate the position of the IV line and the patient's extremity.

Do not forcefully irrigate an apparently occluded line.

KEY TERM

Thromboembolism—obstruction of a blood vessel by a thrombus that is detached from its site.

Infection. Any invasive procedure can result in infection. The judicious use of aseptic technique can minimize the risk of infection. The prehospital environment sometimes imposes less than optimal conditions for maintaining asepsis, but every attempt should be made to do so.

Infiltration. Infiltration occurs when fluid leaks into the tissue surrounding the vein. This can result from a displaced needle or catheter or from fluid leaking from a damaged vein. Infiltration can occur acutely and may be observed in the field. It is evidenced by pain, swelling, and discoloration near the insertion site. Should infiltration occur, the IV should be discontinued and restarted in another site, preferably the opposite arm. If the same arm is used, the vein selected must be proximal to the infiltrated area.

Circulatory (fluid volume) overload. Circulatory, or fluid volume overload can result from fluid being infused too rapidly. It can occur acutely. All patients receiving IV fluids should be continuously monitored for signs and symptoms of circulatory overload. These include distended neck veins; weak and rapid pulse; rapid, shallow respirations; fine auscultatory crackles; dyspnea; and edema.

Catheter shearing. Although catheter shearing is a rare complication of IV therapy, it can have serious consequences. Catheter shearing occurs when all or a portion of the catheter is severed or breaks loose and is free floating. The catheter may move and occlude some part of the venous circulation. The management of catheter shearing requires angiography to retrieve the catheter.

Administering IV Medications

IV medications are given in two ways: IV push (IVP) or IV piggyback (IVPB). IVP refers to the administration of a drug directly into a vein or an established line (primary IV). Medications are usually given through an established IV line, but they may be given by direct injection into a vein, using a needle and syringe. IV medications may be injected either over a specific period of time or administered rapidly as a bolus. An IVPB refers to the administration of IV medication by adding the medication to a bag or bottle of fluid and attaching (piggybacking) it to an already established IV line.

Before administering any drug intravenously, paramedics must be aware of certain points of information. These include dilution, compatibility, and rate of administration.

Most medications used in the prehospital setting come prepackaged in prepared syringes that require no dilution. Some medications, however, are available in vials or ampules and require dilution in a specific amount of fluid prior to being administered. Examples of IV medications that must be diluted prior to administration are isoproterenol and dopamine hydrochloride.

Compatibility of drugs means that one drug can safely be given with another drug at the same time and through the same route with no loss of effectiveness or harmful effects. IV medications must be compatible with the fluid used for dilution as well as with the fluid in the primary IV. If different drugs are being administered through the same line, their compatibility must be confirmed. For example, epinephrine should not be administered at the same time as sodium bicarbonate.

Some drugs have a specific rate for administration. Administering the drug any faster can cause serious side effects. Examples of such drugs are phenytoin and aminophylline.

Administering an IV push

1. Explain the procedure to the patient.
2. Wash hands; don gloves.
3. Prepare the medication.
4. Check patency of the primary line by aspirating gently and noting for blood return.
5. Cleanse the medication port (generally the port closest to the patient should be used).
6. Insert the needle into the medication port (Figure 3-52).

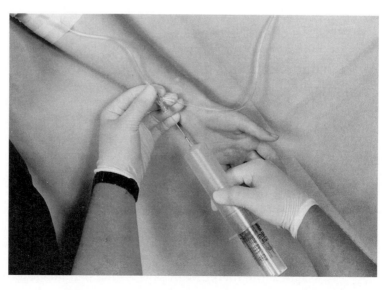

Figure 3-52   Insert needle into the medication port.

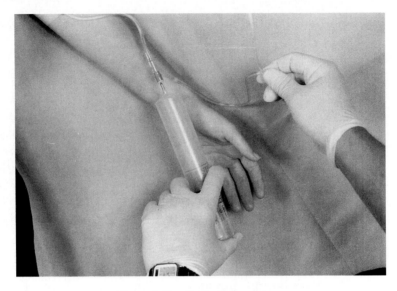

Figure 3-53   Occlude the tubing.

7. Occlude the tubing above the injection port by using the roller clamp or crimping the tube with the other hand (Figure 3-53).
8. Administer the medication at the appropriate rate.
9. Remove the needle and dispose of it properly.
10. Open the roller clamp and release the tubing.
11. Readjust the flow rate.
12. Document the date, time, and amount of drug administered.
13. Assess the patient's response to the drug.

Administering an IV piggyback
1. Explain the procedure to the patient.
2. Wash hands; don gloves.
3. Prepare the medication.
4. Cleanse the injection port on the bag of fluid being used for the IVPB (Figure 3-54).
5. Inject the medication into the bag of fluid (Figure 3-55).
6. Attach a medication label to the bag indicating the name and amount of drug injected.
7. Insert the solution set as usual. Apply a needle (18- to 20-gauge) to the distal end of the tubing.
8. Check patency of the primary line.
9. Cleanse the medication port of the primary tubing.
10. Insert the needle into the injection port and secure with tape.

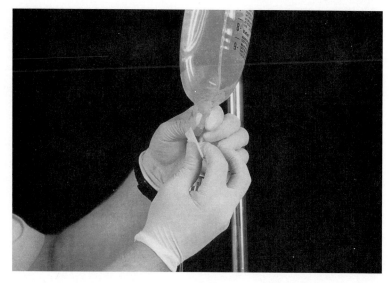

Figure 3-54   Cleanse the injection port.

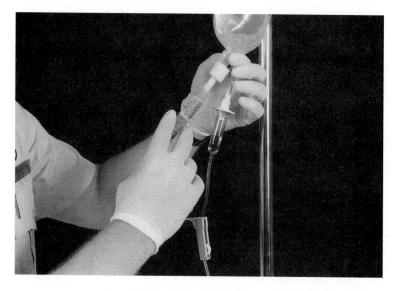

Figure 3-55   Inject medication into bag.

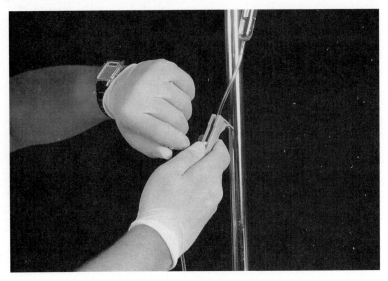

Figure 3-56   Adjust flow rate.

11. Adjust the flow rate (Figure 3-56). The primary line may be clamped off at this point or both bags of fluid may be infused simultaneously.

INTRAOSSEOUS INFUSION

Establishing IV access in pediatric patients can be difficult and time consuming in the emergency setting.[9, 11, 12] A widely used method in the 1950s, intraosseous (IO) infusion has regained popularity as an alternative route for the emergency administration of drugs and fluids, particularly in children. The IO route is intended for short-term use until other venous access can be obtained and should be reserved for serious emergencies, such as cardiopulmonary arrest, shock, extensive burns, and major trauma.[8, 10, 12] Although the technique can be used in older children and adults, it is generally used in children less than 3 years of age.[8, 9]

How it Works

The distribution of fluids and drugs given via the IO route is similar to that of IV administration.[8] The IO route utilizes the vascular network of the long bones (Figure 3-57). Fluids or medications are injected into the bone marrow cavity and pass into the venous sinusoids to the central venous channels and then to systemic circulation via the emissary and nutrient vein.

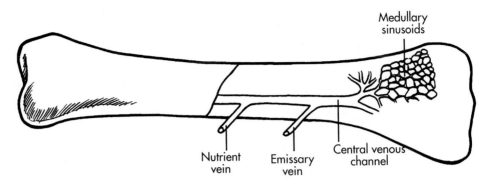

Figure 3-57 Vascular network of long bones.

Advantages and Disadvantages

The IO route offers several advantages. The insertion technique is easily learned and can be accomplished rapidly.[5] In one study, 15 attempts at IO insertion by paramedics in 13 children resulted in all intraosseous needles being placed in less than 30 seconds.[11] The agents that can be administered intraosseously are not limited as with other routes (e.g., endotracheal, sublingual, or rectal). Drugs, fluids (e.g., crystalloids and 50% dextrose in water), electrolytes, and even whole blood can be successfully administered by this route.[8]

Insertion Sites

The insertion sites for IO infusion commonly used today are the proximal tibia, distal tibia, and distal femur. The proximal tibia is used most frequently because it has a broad, flat surface and little muscle or soft tissue overlying it. The site of insertion is 1 to 2 finger breadths (1 to 3 cm) below the tibial tuberosity on the anteromedial surface of the bone (Figure 3-58). Use of the proximal tibia is limited to infants and young children.[12]

The distal tibia also provides an excellent site for IO infusion. The site of insertion is in the medial surface of the tibia 1 to 3 cm above the medial malleolus (Figure 3-59). The distal femur is selected less frequently because the overlying muscle and fat make identifying the site of insertion difficult. The insertion site is 3 cm superior to the lateral condyle of the knee (Figure 3-60).

Equipment

The fluid, tubing, and solution administration sets for IO infusion are the same as those used for IV therapy. Additional equipment includes a

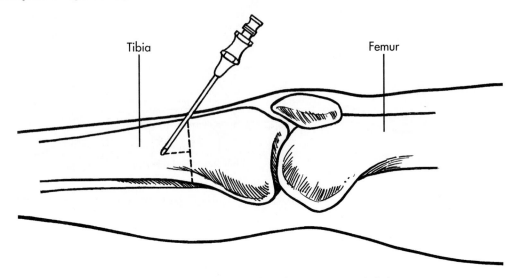

Figure 3-58   Proximal tibial site for intraosseous infusion.

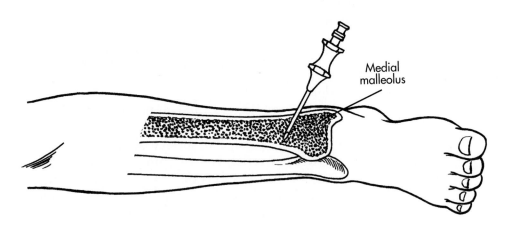

Figure 3-59   Distal tibial site for intraosseous infusion.

three-way stopcock, pressure pump, and a needle with a stylet. Although most spinal needles or bone marrow needles can be used, needles specifically designed for IO infusion are available (Figure 3-61). An 18- to 20-gauge needle can be used in children less than 18 months of age and a 13- to 16-gauge needle is suitable for older children.[12]

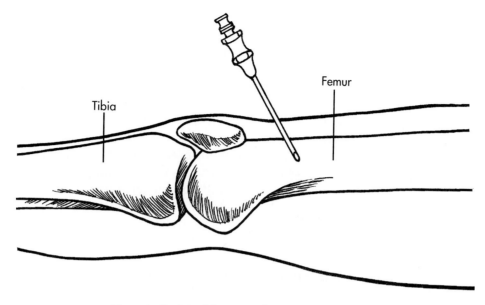

Figure 3-60   Distal femur site for intraosseous infusion.

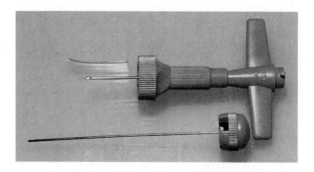

Figure 3-61   Intraosseous needle.

Procedure

1. Explain the procedure to the patient.
2. Wash hands; don gloves.
3. Prepare fluid.
4. Identify the insertion site.
5. Cleanse the site.

6. Insert the needle at a 90-degree angle to the surface of the bone, angled slightly away from the joint. Insertion of the needle should be made with a screwing or boring motion until the bone marrow cavity is penetrated. Penetration of the bone marrow cavity is characterized by a sudden lack of resistance.
7. Remove the stylet.
8. Check needle placement. The needle is determined to be placed properly when (a) bone marrow can be aspirated into a saline-filled syringe, (b) saline can be infused without resistance or sign of infiltration, or (c) the needle stands without support.
9. Connect the IV tubing and administer fluid.
10. Secure the needle with bulky dressing.

Infusion Rates

Fluid should infuse by gravity, but the rate may be unacceptably slow for fluid resuscitation. To improve the infusion rate pressure can be applied to the bag, or a three-way stopcock can be placed in the line and a syringe can be used to push the fluid in.

Although IO administration is relatively complication-free, cases of infection (osteomyelitis) and tibial fracture have been reported. Extravasation of fluid can occur if the needle becomes dislodged or penetrates the entire diameter of the bone.

Contraindications

Insertion of IV lines should be avoided in a recently fractured bone or in the presence of infection or injury to the tissue overlying the bone.

AGE-RELATED CONCERNS

There are several issues related to the administration of medication in pediatric and elderly patients. Three major concerns in administering drugs to these two groups of patients are adequate muscle size, difficulty of establishing IV access, and need for adjusting dosages based on body weight or other physiologic attributes.

Pediatric Patients

Drugs should be administered to children in the most nonthreatening manner possible. Paramedics should attempt to gain the cooperation of the child by simple and truthful explanations. It is usually helpful to allow the parent to hold the child and assist with the procedure.

Although the principles and techniques of pediatric parenteral drug administration are similar to those for adults, there are special considerations for the administration of IM injections in young patients. The younger the child, the less muscle mass available for injection. Selection criteria of the appropriate site for IM injection in children are shown in Table 3-4. To provide adequate safety children should be restrained for injections. The preferred needle size for pediatric intramuscular injections are 25- to 27-gauge and ½ to 1 inch in length.

Drug doses in children are usually ordered according to the body weight or surface area of the child. Formulas for calculating doses in children are provided in Chapter 4.

Geriatric Patients

In elderly patients drug absorption and distribution with SC and IM administration are slowed because circulation may be diminished by aging and illnesses, such as congestive heart failure (see Chapter 2). IV administration is therefore particularly important in managing emergencies in elderly patients. IV access can be as much a challenge in the very old as it is in the very young. It may be necessary for paramedics to select smaller IV catheters (e.g., 20-gauge) than those used with younger adults.

When IM injections are given to elderly patients, sites should be selected carefully. Muscle mass decreases with age, decreasing the number of suitable sites for injections. Muscles should be palpated carefully to ensure adequate size, and the muscle should be pinched up.

Table 3-4 Selection of Appropriate Intramuscular Injection Sites in Children

SITE	APPROPRIATENESS
Deltoid	Not used for children under 5 years of age; muscle should be pinched up rather than pulled taut
Vastis lateralis	Preferred site for children under 3 years of age
Dorsogluteal	Should not be used for injections in children under 4 years of age if other IM sites are available
Ventrogluteal	Preferred site for children over 3 years of age who have been walking for at least 1 year

SUMMARY

Paramedics must develop safe practices and habits for drug administration. Safety for oneself, fellow crewmembers, and patients should always be the highest priority for paramedics, and this is equally true in drug therapy.

Patient safety in drug therapy is best ensured by guaranteeing the five rights: right patient, right drug, right dose, right route, and right time. The benefit of prompt, safe administration of drugs in the field include life-saving treatment, as well as improved patient comfort and relief of pain. Errors in drug therapy, however, can result in significant harm to patients and even death.

Safety concerns with drug administration include appropriate handling of sharps and infectious disposables to prevent the risk of exposure to bloodborne pathogens.

REFERENCES

1. Aitkenhead AR: Drug administration during CPR: what route? *Resuscitation,* 22(2):191, 1991.
2. Crespo SG et al: Comparison of two doses of endotracheal epinephrine in a cardiac arrest model, *Ann Emerg Med* 20(3):230, 1991.
3. Drawbaugh RE, Deibler CG, Eitel DR: Prehospital administration of rectal diazepam in pediatric status epilepticus, *Prehosp Disast Med* 5(2):155, 1990.
4. Friery J, Weiner K: Start an IV in that bone, *Emergency* 9(11):28, 1987.
5. Fuch S, Lacovey D, Paris P: Intraosseous infusion in the prehospital setting, *Prehosp Disast Med* 4(1):80, 1989 (abstract).
6. Mace SE: Differences in plasma lidocaine levels with drug therapy secondary to total volume of diluent administered, *Resuscitation* 20(3):185, 1990.
7. Orlowski JP, Gallagher JM, Porembka DT: Endotracheal epinephrine is unreliable, *Resuscitation* 19(2):103, 1990.
8. Peck KR, Altieri M: Intraosseous infusions: an old technique with modern applications, *Pediatr Nurs* 14(4):296, 1988.
9. Rositti VA et al: Intraosseous infusion: an alternative route of pediatric intravascular access, *Ann Emerg Med* 103, September 1985.
10. Simon JE, Goldberg AT: *Prehospital Pediatric Life Support,* St Louis, 1989, Mosby–Year Book.
11. Smith RJ et al: Intraosseous infusion by prehospital personnel in critically ill pediatric patients, *Ann Emerg Med* 17(5):97, 1988.
12. Spivey WH: Intraosseous infusions, *J Pediatr* 111(5):639, 1987.
13. Stroup CA: Intraosseous infusion: prehospital use in the critically ill pediatric patient, *J Emerg Med Serv* 12(5):38, 1987.
14. West K: Assessing the risks, *Emergency* 24(3):30, 1992.

4

Dose Calculation

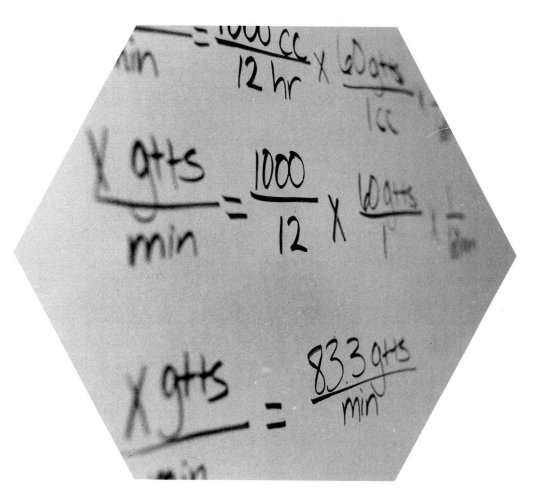

OBJECTIVES

1. List three units of measurement for volume, linear, and weight measurement.
2. State the meanings of common metric prefixes.
3. Demonstrate conversion of values among systems of measurement.
4. Discuss the advantages of the dimensional analysis method of dose calculations.
5. Calculate doses using the basic formula.
6. Calculate doses using dimensional analysis.

Paramedics are often required to translate a physician's drug order into the accurate volume of the drug or fluid they are administering. This includes accurately calculating IV drip rates. Although these calculations are usually a matter of simple arithmetic, they can also be complex. Thus it is necessary to understand systems of measurement, to be able to convert between systems of measurement, and to calculate doses. In this chapter two methods of calculation are presented: the basic formula and the dimensional analysis.

SYSTEMS OF MEASUREMENT

Three systems of measurement are used in the United States: metric, apothecary, and household. The metric system has been adopted internationally and is the most widely used. It is also considered the most convenient of the three systems because it is a decimal system based on units that are factors of 10. The basic units are the meter (linear measurement), the liter (volume measurement), and the gram (weight measurement).

Table 4-1 Common Metric Prefixes and Meanings

PREFIX	MEANING
kilo-	1000 times greater
deci-	10 times less
centi-	100 times less
milli-	1000 times less
micro-	1,000,000 times less

These basic units can be divided into 10, 100, or 1000 parts, or can be multiplied by 10, 100, or 1000 to form secondary units. The names of these secondary units are formed by adding Greek or Latin prefixes to the basic units. For example, a kilogram is 1000 grams, and a milliliter is 1 one-thousandth of a liter. Table 4-1 lists common metric prefixes and their meanings. Because the metric system is so widely used in health-care settings, the paramedic should become familiar with it. For documentation purposes the National Bureau of Standards International System of Units notation style should be followed (see box below).

INTERNATIONAL SYSTEM OF UNITS NOTATION STYLE

1. Periods should not be used with abbreviations of units (kg, not k.g. or kg.).
2. Units are not capitalized (kilogram, not Kilogram).
3. A single space is placed between the number and the unit abbreviation (10 kg, not 10kg).
4. Abbreviations are not pluralized (kg, not kgs).
5. Fractions are not used with metric units of measurement (0.50 mg, not 1/2 mg).
6. Values less than 1 should have a zero to the left of the decimal for metric units of measurement (0.25 mg not .25 mg).

Table 4-2 Systems of Measurement: Abbreviations and Symbols

METRIC	HOUSEHOLD	APOTHECARY
Length	**Length**	
meter = m	inch = in	
centimeter = cm	foot = ft	
millimeter = mm		
Volume	**Volume**	**Volume**
liter = L	drops = gtt	minim = ℳ
milliliter = ml	teaspoon = tsp or t	fluid dram = fl dr
cubic centimeter = cc	tablespoon = tbsp or T	fluid ounce = fl oz
	ounce = oz	
	cup = c	
	pint = p	
	quart = q	
	gallon = gal	
Weight	**Weight**	**Weight**
kilogram = kg	pound = lb	grain = gr
gram = g	ounce = oz	dram = dr
milligram = mg		
microgram = μg		

The apothecary system is an old system of measurement used by pharmacists (apothecaries) in colonial America. The basic units of this system are the minim (volume) and the grain (weight). The apothecary system is gradually being phased out, but some of its units, such as the pound, are still widely used.

The household method is a system of measurement commonly used in the home. The household units for weight are ounces and pounds. The household units for volume are teaspoons, tablespoons, cups, pints, quarts, and gallons. The household system is not widely used, except in the home. Both the apothecary system and the household system are less precise than the metric system. Each system has its own symbols and abbreviations (Table 4-2).

CONVERSION

Because all three systems of measurement are used in the United States, one of the most important skills in accurate dose calculation is the ability to convert given values from one system to another. Generally, the conversions required for dose calculation are from the household or apothecary systems to the metric system (as in pounds to kilograms), or from unit to unit within the metric system (grams to milligrams). The need for conversion is frequently encountered when a drug dose is ordered based on a patient's weight. For example, dopamine administration is based on a patient's weight in kilograms. The patient's weight is usually given in pounds, so it is necessary to convert pounds to kilograms before proceeding with the dose calculation.

One unit of measure can be converted to another by using a **conversion factor**. Although it may be helpful to memorize a few key equivalencies (conversion factors), it is generally best to have a chart with this information readily available (Tables 4-3 and 4-4). Once the appropriate conversion factor has been determined, it is multiplied by the original value to find the answer. *Remember: Fractions are not used in the metric system, so the answer is converted to decimal form.*

KEY TERM

Conversion factor—an equivalent numerical value that produces a change in the form of a quantity without changing its value.

Table 4-3   Conversion Factors/Equivalents

METRIC	APOTHECARY	HOUSEHOLD
1 ml	15–16 m	
4–5 ml	1 fl dr	1 t
15–16 ml	3–4 fl dr	1 T
30–32 ml	1 fl oz	2 T
240 ml	8 fl oz	1 c
500 ml	16 fl oz	1 pt
1,000 ml	32 fl oz	1 qt
60 mg	1 gr	
1 g	15–16 gr	
4 g	1 dr	
1 kg		2.2 lb
2.54 cm		1 in

Table 4-4   Commonly Used Conversion Factors (Quick Reference)

5 ml	=	1	t
15 ml	=	1	T
30 ml	=	1	oz
1 mg	=	1000	μg
1 g	=	1000	mg
1 kg	=	1000	g
1 kg	=	2.2	lb
1 ml	=	1	cc
1 L	=	1000	ml

EXAMPLES

Example #1: In this example it is necessary to convert grains (apothecary system) to milligrams (metric system).

How many milligrams are equal to 5 gr?

Step 1

State the problem, beginning with the desired unit of measure.

x mg = 5 gr

Step 2

Identify the conversion factor and place it in the equation. The **numerator** of the conversion factor must be the same as the unit of the desired answer.

$$x \text{ mg} = 5 \text{ gr} \times \frac{60 \text{ mg}}{1 \text{ gr}}$$

Step 3

Cancel like units that appear on the same side of the equation.

$$x \text{ mg} = 5 \text{ g̶r̶} \times \frac{60 \text{ mg}}{1 \text{ g̶r̶}}$$

Step 4

Complete the mathematical operations.

$$x \text{ mg} = \frac{5 \times 60 \text{ mg}}{1} = \frac{300 \text{ mg}}{1}$$

Answer = 300 mg

Example #2: In this example it is necessary to convert pounds (apothecary) to kilograms (metric).

Mr. Smith gives his weight as 188 lb. How many kilograms does he weigh? (Conversion factor: 2.2 lb = 1 kg)

Step 1

State the problem, beginning with the desired unit of measure.

$$x \text{ kg} = 188 \text{ lb}$$

Step 2

Identify the conversion factor and place it in the equation. The numerator of the conversion factor must be the same as the unit of the desired answer.

$$x \text{ kg} = 188 \text{ lb} \times \frac{1 \text{ kg}}{2.2 \text{ lb}}$$

KEY TERM

Numerator—the term of a fraction above or to the left of the line that expresses the number of parts of a unit.

Step 3

Cancel like units that appear on the same side of the equation.

$$x \text{ kg} = 188 \cancel{\text{lb}} \times \frac{1 \text{ kg}}{2.2 \cancel{\text{lb}}}$$

Step 4

Complete the mathematical operations.

$$x \text{ kg} = \frac{188 \times 1 \text{ kg}}{2.2} = \frac{188}{2.2} \text{ kg}$$

Answer = 85.45 kg

SELF TEST

Using the conversion chart, work the following conversion problems. Answers appear in Appendix C

1. _____ mg = gr x
2. _____ gr = 100 mg
3. _____ mg = gr $\frac{1}{150}$
4. _____ kg = 190 lb
5. _____ cm = 4 in

6. _____ lb = 40 kg
7. _____ mg = 3 g
8. _____ L = 500 ml
9. _____ mg = 1.5 kg
10. _____ g = 900 mg

CALCULATION METHODS

Several different methods of dose calculation exist, the most common ones being ratio and proportion, basic formula, and dimensional analysis. The authors recommend that the student become comfortable with one system and use it exclusively. This chapter discusses and gives examples of the basic formula and dimensional analysis.

Basic Formula

The basic formula, also called "dose on hand," is a popular calculation method, probably because it is so easy to recall. The basic formula has traditionally been used in the prehospital setting. Use of this method requires the memorization of a formula and the conversion of all components to like units before inserting them into the formula:

$$\frac{D \text{ (desired dose)} \times V \text{ (vehicle—e.g., tablet, liquid)}}{H \text{ (dose on hand)}} = \text{amount to give}$$

or:

$$\frac{D \times V}{H}$$

where D is the drug dose that has been ordered by the physician, H is the concentration in which the drug is supplied, V is the form and amount in which the drug is supplied. This may be expressed as volume (ml) or in tablets, capsules, etc. In emergency medicine it is most commonly expressed as volume.

To solve calculation problems using the basic formula:

1. Convert units of measurement to the same system (metric, apothecary, or household) and the same unit of measurement.
2. Insert the given numbers into the equation.
3. Solve the problem, canceling units when possible and reducing by dividing the numerator and **denominator** by a common number.

EXAMPLES

Example #1: Order   Demerol 50 mg IM
              On hand   Demerol 75 mg/1 ml
How many milliliters should be administered?

Step 1

No conversion is necessary.

Step 2

Insert numbers into the equation.

$$\frac{50 \text{ mg (D)} \times 1 \text{ ml (V)}}{75 \text{ mg (H)}}$$

Step 3

Solve the problem. (Step continued on next page.)

KEY TERM

Denominator—divisor; the term of a fraction that expresses the number of equal parts into which a unit is divided; the denominator appears below or to the right of the line.

$$\frac{50 \text{ mg/ml}}{75 \text{ mg}} = \frac{50 \text{ ml}}{75} = 0.66 \text{ ml (round to 0.7 ml)}$$

Example #2: Order   Valium 5 mg IV push
              On hand   Valium 10 mg/1 ml
How many milliliters should be administered?

Step 1

No conversion is necessary.

Step 2

Insert numbers into the equation.

$$\frac{5 \text{ mg (D)} \times 1 \text{ ml (V)}}{10 \text{ mg (H)}}$$

Step 3

Solve the problem.

$$\frac{5 \text{ mg/ml}}{10 \text{ mg}} = \frac{1 \text{ ml}}{2} = 0.5 \text{ ml}$$

Example #3: Order   furosemide 10 mg IV push
              On hand   furosemide 40 mg/4 ml
How many milliliters should be administered?

Step 1

No conversion is necessary.

Step 2

Insert numbers into the equation.

$$\frac{10 \text{ mg (D)} \times 4 \text{ ml (V)}}{40 \text{ mg (H)}}$$

Step 3

Solve the problem.

$$\frac{40 \text{ mg/ml}}{40 \text{ mg}} = \frac{1 \text{ ml}}{1} = 1 \text{ ml}$$

Example #4: Order   morphine sulfate 4 mg
              On hand   morphine sulfate ⅙ gr per ml
How many milliliters should be administered?

Step 1

Convert grains to milligrams.

$$\frac{60\ mg}{1\ gr} \times \frac{1\ gr}{6} = \frac{60\ mg}{6} = 10\ mg$$

Step 2

Insert numbers into the equation.

$$\frac{4\ mg\ (D) \times 1\ ml\ (V)}{10\ mg\ (H)}$$

Step 3

Solve the problem.

$$\frac{4\ mg/ml}{10\ mg} = \frac{4\ ml}{10} = 0.4\ ml$$

The basic formula method is easy to remember and used for many types of calculations. However, when calculations become more complex and require multiple conversions and mathematical operations, a method called dimensional analysis is more practical.

Dimensional Analysis

The dimensional analysis method is actually based on the same principles as simple conversions and the basic formula. Unlike the basic formula, however, there is no formula to memorize. All the conversion factors are set up in one equation and separated by multiplication signs.

To solve calculation problems using a dimensional analysis equation:

1. Set up the equation. The unit of measurement desired in the answer (ml, mg, drops per minute, etc.) is placed to the left of the equal sign. The first factor is placed to the right of the equal sign and is the same unit as the answer.
2. Cancel pairs of units of measure (labels) that appear in numerator and denominator. For components that are not ratios the number is placed over 1 without the unit label. The only unit remaining after cancellation should be the unit of the answer. *If this does not occur, the equation is set up incorrectly.* (This is a unique feature of dimensional analysis and one that proves to be an advantage over other calculation techniques.) At the same time, reduce the fractions by dividing both numerators and denominators by a common number.

3. Multiply the numerators.
4. Multiply the denominators.
5. Divide the numerator by the denominator.

EXAMPLES

Example #1: Order Demerol   50 mg IM stat
             On hand Demerol   75 mg/1 ml
How many milliliters should be administered?

Step 1

Set up the equation. The unit of measure desired in the answer is placed to the left of the equal sign. The first factor is the same unit as the answer.

$$ml = \frac{1\ ml}{75\ mg} \times \frac{50\ mg}{1}$$

Step 2

Cancel like units and evenly divisible numbers. If the remaining unit is that of the answer, the problem is set up correctly.

$$ml = \frac{1\ ml}{75\ \cancel{mg}} \times \frac{50\ \cancel{mg}}{1}$$

Step 3

Multiply numerators first and then denominators.

$$ml = \frac{1\ ml}{3} \times \frac{2}{1}$$

Step 4

Divide the numerator by the denominator.

$$ml = \frac{2}{3} = .66\ ml\ (\text{round to } 0.7\ ml)$$

Example #2: Order   Valium 5 mg IV push
             On hand   Valium 10 mg/1 ml
How many milliliters should be administered?

Step 1

Set up the equation.

$$ml = \frac{1\ ml}{10\ mg} \times \frac{5\ mg}{1}$$

Step 2

Cancel like units and evenly divisible numbers.

$$\text{ml} = \frac{1 \text{ ml}}{10 \text{ mg}} \times \frac{5 \text{ mg}}{1}$$

Step 3

Multiply numerators first and then denominators.

$$\text{ml} = \frac{1 \text{ ml}}{2 \text{ mg}} \times \frac{1 \text{ mg}}{1}$$

Step 4

Divide the numerator by the denominator.

$$\text{ml} = \frac{1 \text{ ml}}{2} = .50 \text{ ml}$$

Example #3: Order   furosemide 10 mg IV push
                 On hand   furosemide 40 mg/4 ml
How many milliliters should be administered?

Step 1

Set up the equation.

$$\text{ml} = \frac{4 \text{ ml}}{40 \text{ mg}} \times \frac{10 \text{ mg}}{1}$$

Step 2

Cancel like units and evenly divisible numbers.

$$\text{ml} = \frac{4 \text{ ml}}{40 \text{ mg}} \times \frac{10 \text{ mg}}{1}$$

Step 3

Multiply numerators first and then denominators.

$$\text{ml} = \frac{4 \text{ ml}}{4} \times \frac{1}{1}$$

Step 4

Divide the numerator by the denominator.

$$\text{ml} = \frac{4 \text{ ml}}{4} = 1 \text{ ml}$$

Example #4: Order   morphine sulfate 4 mg
              On hand   morphine sulfate ⅙ gr/ml

How many milliliters should be administered?

Step 1

Set up the equation.

$$ml = \frac{ml}{\frac{1}{6}\ gr} \times \frac{1\ gr}{60\ mg} \times \frac{4\ mg}{1}$$

Step 2

Cancel like units and evenly divisible numbers.

$$ml = \frac{ml}{\frac{1}{6}\ \cancel{gr}} \times \frac{1\ \cancel{gr}}{60\ \cancel{mg}} \times \frac{4\ \cancel{mg}}{1}$$

Step 3

Multiply numerators first and then denominators.

$$ml = \frac{4\ ml}{\frac{1}{6} \times 60} = \frac{4\ ml}{10}$$

Step 4

Divide the numerator by the denominator.

$$ml = \frac{4\ ml}{10} = 0.4\ ml$$

Different kinds of calculation problems can be set up in the same fashion, including IV drip rate calculations, oral and parenteral doses, and titrated doses based on body weight.

CALCULATION OF IV DRIP RATES

When administering fluids, the paramedic must calculate the rate in gtt per minute at which the fluid should be administered. To calculate drip rates the following information is necessary to set up the equation:

- Amount to be administered
- Period of time for administration
- Drop factor (number of drops per milliliter for a given infusion set)

Sometimes the conversion factor 1 hr = 60 min is also necessary.

EXAMPLES

Example #1: Order   250 ml normal saline over 90 min
              Infusion set delivers 10 gtt/ml
Calculate gtt/min.

Step 1

Set up the equation.

$$\frac{gtt}{min} = \frac{10 \ gtt}{1 \ ml} \times \frac{250 \ ml}{90 \ min}$$

Step 2

Cancel like units and evenly divisible numbers.

$$\frac{gtt}{min} = \frac{10 \ gtt}{1 \ \cancel{ml}} \times \frac{250 \ \cancel{ml}}{90 \ min}$$

Step 3

Multiply numerators first and then denominators.

$$\frac{gtt}{min} = \frac{2500 \ gtt}{90 \ min}$$

Step 4

Divide the numerator by the denominator.

$$\frac{gtt}{min} = 27.77 \ (\text{round to } 28) = 28 \ gtt/min$$

Example #2: Order   1000 ml D$_5$W over 6 hr
              Infusion set delivers 15 gtt/ml
How many gtt/min should be administered?

Step 1

Set up the equation.

$$\frac{gtt}{min} = \frac{15 \ gtt}{1 \ ml} \times \frac{1000 \ ml}{6 \ hr} \times \frac{1 \ hr}{60 \ min}$$

Step 2

Cancel like units and evenly divisible numbers.

$$\frac{gtt}{min} = \frac{15 \ gtt}{1 \ \cancel{ml}} \times \frac{1000 \ \cancel{ml}}{6 \ \cancel{hr}} \times \frac{1 \ \cancel{hr}}{60 \ min}$$

Step 3

Multiply numerators first and then denominators.

$$\frac{gtt}{min} = \frac{15 \times 1000}{360} = \frac{15,000}{360}$$

Step 4

Divide the numerator by the denominator.

$$\frac{gtt}{min} = 41.07 \text{ gtt/min} = 41 \text{ gtt/min}$$

Example #3: Order   Dopamine 400 mg in 500 ml D₅W
Administer at a rate of 6 mg/kg/min, mixing two 200 mg ampules of Dopamine in 500 ml D₅W
Drop factor: 60 gtt = 1 ml
Patient weighs 185 lb

Step 1

Set up the equation.

$$\frac{x \text{ gtt}}{min} = \frac{60 \text{ gtt}}{1 \text{ ml}} \times \frac{500 \text{ ml}}{400 \text{ mg}} \times \frac{1 \text{ mg}}{1000 \text{ μg}} \times \frac{6 \text{ μg}}{kg \times min} \times \frac{1 \text{ kg}}{2.2 \text{ lb}} \times \frac{185 \text{ lb}}{1}$$

Step 2

Cancel like units and evenly divisible numbers.

$$\frac{x \text{ gtt}}{min} = \frac{60 \text{ gtt}}{1 \text{ ml}} \times \frac{500 \text{ ml}}{400 \text{ mg}} \times \frac{1 \text{ mg}}{1000 \text{ μg}} \times \frac{6 \text{ μg}}{kg \times min} \times \frac{1 \text{ kg}}{2.2 \text{ lb}} \times \frac{185 \text{ lb}}{1}$$

Step 3

Multiply numerators first and then denominators.

$$\frac{x \text{ gtt}}{min} = \frac{3,330 \text{ gtt}}{88 \text{ min}}$$

Step 4

Divide the numerator by the denominator.

$$\frac{37.8 \text{ gtt}}{min} = \frac{38 \text{ gtt}}{min}$$

Note that the only factors left after cancellation of like labels are gtt per minute, which formed the problem.

Example #4: Administer lidocaine intravenously at a rate of 2 mg/min, mixing 2 g lidocaine in 500 ml D_5W

Drop factor = 60 gtts/1 ml

How many gtt per minute should be administered?

Step 1

Set up the equation.

$$\frac{x \text{ gtt}}{\text{min}} = \frac{60 \text{ gtt}}{\text{ml}} \times \frac{500 \text{ ml}}{2 \text{ g}} \times \frac{1 \text{ g}}{1000 \text{ mg}} \times \frac{2 \text{ mg}}{\text{min}}$$

Step 2

Cancel like units and evenly divisible numbers.

$$\frac{x \text{ gtt}}{\text{min}} = \frac{60 \text{ gtt}}{\cancel{\text{ml}}} \times \frac{500 \cancel{\text{ml}}}{2 \cancel{\text{g}}} \times \frac{1 \cancel{\text{g}}}{1000 \cancel{\text{mg}}} \times \frac{2 \cancel{\text{mg}}}{\text{min}}$$

Step 3

Multiply numerators first and then denominators.

$$\frac{x \text{ gtt}}{\text{min}} = \frac{60 \text{ gtt}}{2 \text{ min}}$$

Step 4

Divide the numerator by the denominator.

$$\frac{30 \text{ gtt}}{\text{min}}$$

SELF TEST

Calculate the following dose problems using the dimensional analysis system. Answers and work for these problems appear in Appendix C.

1. Order: morphine sulfate 2 mg IV push
   On hand: morphine sulfate 10 mg/ml. Dilute the morphine in 9 ml normal saline to equal 1 mg/ml
   How many milliliters will you administer?
2. Order: 12 mg adenosine IV push
   On hand: adenosine 6 mg/2 ml
   How many milliliters will you administer?
3. Order: bretylium 5 mg/kg
   On hand: bretylium 500 mg in 10 ml

Patient weighs 242 lb
How many milliliters will you administer?

4. Order: epinephrine 1 μg/min
   On hand: 1 mg diluted in 250 ml D$_5$W
   Administration set delivers 60 gtt/ml
   How many gtt per minute will you deliver?

5. Order: Demerol 35 mg IV push
   On hand: Demerol 50 mg/ml
   How many milliliters will you administer?

6. Order: oxytocin 5 units IM
   On hand: oxytocin 10 units/ml
   How many milliliters will you administer?

7. Order: Ringer's lactate 300 ml over 30 min
   On hand: Ringer's lactate 1000 ml
   Administration set delivers 10 gtt/ml
   How many gtt per minute will you administer?

8. Order: furosemide 60 mg IV push
   On hand: furosemide 20 mg/2 ml
   How many milliliters will you administer?

9. Order: atropine 0.5 mg IV push
   On hand: atropine 1 mg/ml
   How many milliliters will you administer?

10. Order: isoproterenol 4 μg/min via IV infusion
    On hand: 1 mg isoproterenol per 250 ml D$_5$W
    Administration set delivers 60 gtt/ml
    How many gtt per minute will you administer?

11. Order: Normal saline 1000 ml over 4 hr
    On hand: Normal saline 1000 ml
    Administration set delivers 15 gtt/ml
    How many gtt per minute will you administer?

12. Order: dobutamine 8 μg/kg/min via IV infusion
    On hand: dobutamine 250 mg in 250 ml D$_5$W
    Administration set delivers 60 gtt/ml
    Patient weighs 198 lb
    How many milliliters per hour will the patient receive?

13. Order: dopamine 6 μg/kg/min via IV infusion
    On hand: dopamine 400 mg in 500 ml D$_5$W
    Administration set delivers 60 gtt/ml
    Patient weighs 90 kg
    Determine the rate of infusion in gtt per minute.

14. Order: lidocaine 2 mg/min via IV infusion
    On hand: lidocaine 2 g in 500 ml D$_5$W

How many milliliters per hour will you administer?

15. Order: dextran 40 250 ml over 90 min
On hand: dextran 40, 500 ml
Administration set delivers 20 gtt/ml
How many gtt per minute will you deliver?

16. Patient is receiving nitroprusside via IV infusion at 1 µg/kg/min. The order is to reduce the rate of infusion to 0.8 µg/kg/min. The concentration of the solution is 200 µg/ml. The patient weighs 220 lb.
   The solution set provides 60 gtt/ml.
   What is the new rate in gtt per minute?

17. The patient is receiving Dopamine at a rate of 25 ml/hr. The concentration of the solution is 200 mg in 250 ml D_5W.
   How many µg/kg/min is this 90-kg person receiving?

18. The patient is receiving aminophylline via IV infusion at 100 ml/30 min. The concentration of the solution is 125 mg aminophylline in 100 ml D_5W.
   How many milligrams per minute is the patient receiving?

19. The patient is receiving morphine sulfate via IV infusion. The concentration of the solution is 100 mg morphine sulfate in 500 ml IV fluid. It is infusing at a rate of 30 ml/hr.
   How many milligrams per hour is the patient receiving?

20. Your patient is receiving a lidocaine drip at 45 gtt/min. The label indicates that 2 g of lidocaine were added to 500 ml D_5W.
   How many milligrams per minute is the patient receiving?
   Administration set delivers 60 gtt/ml.

SUMMARY

Calculating drug doses is an integral part of medication administration. Although there are currently three systems of measurement used in the United States, the metric system is used most commonly. Conversion between and within each of these systems is a necessary skill for paramedics.

This chapter presents two methods of dose calculation: the basic formula and the dimensional analysis. Dimensional analysis, which does not require memorizing a formula, offers several advantages over the basic formula. Drug calculations range from simple to complex. The ability to accurately calculate doses in a timely manner is essential in the prehospital setting.

REFERENCES

1. Madigan KG: *Prehospital emergency drugs pocket reference*, St Louis, 1990, Mosby–Year Book.
2. Smith AJ: *Dosage and solutions calculations the dimensional analysis way*, St Louis, 1989, Mosby–Year Book.
3. Wilson BA, Shannon MT: *A unified approach to dosage calculation*, Norwalk, CT, 1986, Appleton-Century-Crofts.

5
Fluid and Electrolytes

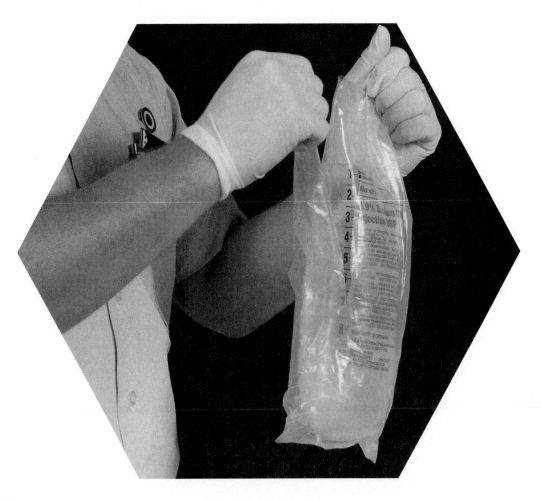

OBJECTIVES

1. Identify the mechanisms by which fluid and electrolyte balance is maintained in the body.
2. Differentiate among hypotonic, isotonic, and hypertonic IV fluids.
3. Define colloid and crystalloid solutions, and give examples of each.
4. List indications for IV fluid therapy in the prehospital setting.
5. Discuss possible side effects of IV fluid therapy.

Fluid and electrolyte balance is essential to the proper functioning of the human body. A basic understanding of this balance is necessary to assess and manage fluid and electrolyte disturbances in the field. This chapter discusses the principles of fluid and electrolyte balance and IV fluid therapy.

FLUID

Body fluids contain water, electrolytes, and other substances. Normally, the volume and composition of body fluid remains relatively constant. Total body fluid comprises approximately 60% of the body weight. The body's fluid is distributed in two principal fluid compartments or spaces: **intracellular** and **extracellular.**

Intracellular fluid (ICF) is located within the cell and consists mostly of water. Three-fourths of all body fluid (comprising 45% of the body weight) is contained in the intracellular space. The remaining fluid is located outside the cell—the extracellular fluid (ECF) compartment.

Extracellular fluid consists of two components: **intravascular** fluid and **interstitial** fluid. Intravascular fluid is found within the blood vessels. Interstitial fluid occupies the space between the cells (outside the cell membrane). Water moves freely between the two fluid compartments.

ELECTROLYTES

An electrolyte is an element or compound that separates into electrically charged particles called ions when dissolved in water. Ions that are negatively charged are called **anions**; positively charged ions are called **cations.** Anions are denoted by a minus sign following their chemical symbol (Cl^-), and cations are denoted by a plus sign (K^+). Table 5-1 lists and

Table 5-1 Major Cations and Anions and Their Functions

CATIONS		ANIONS	
Sodium (Na⁺)	Sodium is the most abundant electrolyte in extracellular fluid. It has a role in the regulation of water distribution. When sodium is lost from the body, water is also lost. Likewise, sodium retention results in water retention. Severe hyponatremia can cause seizures.	**Chloride (Cl⁻)**	Chloride is found primarily in extracellular fluid. There is a reciprocal relationship between the concentrations of chloride and bicarbonate in extracellular fluid. Therefore chloride has a role in acid-base balance.
Potassium (K⁺)	Potassium is the principle cation in intracellular fluid. It plays a crucial role in the formation of electrical impulses in nerves and muscle. It also plays an important role in the initiation of cardiac impulses. Deficits or excesses of potassium can cause serious disturbances in cardiac rhythm.	**Bicarbonate (HCO₃⁻)**	Bicarbonate is the major buffer in the body. It plays a critical role in the maintenance of acid-base balance. Significant losses of bicarbonate result in metabolic acidosis, whereas excesses result in metabolic alkalosis.
Calcium (Ca⁺⁺)	More than 99% of the total body calcium is located in the bones, teeth, and nails. The remaining calcium is in the serum. Calcium plays a major role in bone development, blood clotting, and neuromuscular activity.		
Magnesium (Mg⁺⁺)	Magnesium plays an important role in the metabolism of proteins and carbohydrates and in controlling neuromuscular irritability.		

describes the major anions and cations in extracellular and intracellular fluid.

Electrolytes play a role in: (1) regulating water balance, (2) regulating acid-base balance, (3) enzyme reactions, and (4) neuromuscular activity.[5] Proper balance among the major electrolytes is essential to normal metabolism and function. Electrolytes are measured in **milliequivalents** (mEq).

HOMEOSTASIS

Homeostasis is the body's tendency to maintain a steady state or constant internal environment. Any deficit or excess of fluid or electrolytes can compromise the body's natural balance and adversely affect the health of an individual. Fluids and electrolytes move passively (shift) or are actively transported across cell membranes within the body to maintain physiologic balance. For example, when intravascular fluid is lost (as with hemorrhage), intracellular fluid shifts to the intravascular space to restore fluid balance.

TRANSPORTATION OF FLUID AND ELECTROLYTES

Cell membranes are *semipermeable*, meaning they permit some molecules to cross readily while blocking the passage of others. Generally, small molecules, such as water, cross readily, whereas larger molecules, such as plasma proteins, are restricted. Substances cross the cell membrane by both passive and active transport.

Passive Transport

Passive transport does not require the expenditure of energy. Three means of passive transport are **diffusion**, **filtration**, and **osmosis**.

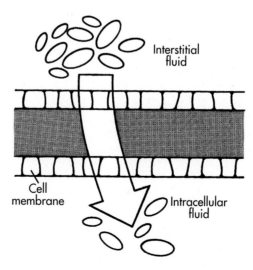

Figure 5-1 Diffusion. Solutes move from an area of high concentration to an area of low concentration.

Diffusion is the movement of **solutes** (molecules or ions in solution) from an area of high concentration to an area of lower concentration (Figure 5-1). The difference in concentration of a particular solute between one side of a semipermeable membrane and the other is referred to as a *gradient*. Generally, solutes diffuse across a semipermeable membrane until the concentration on both sides is equalized.

Filtration is the movement of fluid and electrolytes in response to **hydrostatic pressure** gradients. Substances move from areas of greater pressure to areas of lesser pressure.

Osmosis refers to movement of water (solvent) across semipermeable membranes from areas of low solute concentration to areas of high solute concentration (Figure 5-2). This movement of water is affected by the **tonicity** of the solutions on either side of the cell membrane.

When two solutions are compared, a solution of higher solute concentration is referred to as **hypertonic**. A cell placed in a hypertonic solution would lose water or shrink in size. A solution of lower solute concentration is **hypotonic**. A cell placed in a hypotonic solution would gain water or increase in size. Solutions of equal solute concentration are **isotonic**. A cell placed in an isotonic solution would not change in size (Figure 5-3).

Solutions with solute concentrations equal to that of plasma are considered isotonic solutions. Lactated Ringer's solution and normal saline (0.9% sodium chloride) are examples of isotonic solutions. Hypotonic solutions, such as 0.45% sodium chloride (half normal saline), have solute concentrations less than that of plasma, whereas hypertonic solutions, such as 10% dextrose in water, have solute concentrations higher than that of plasma. Figures 5-4, 5-5, and 5-6 depict the effect of tonicity on the movement of intracellular and interstitial fluid.

Active Transport

Active transport requires the expenditure of energy. It provides for the movement of substances against a concentration gradient. For example,

---

KEY TERMS

Hypertonic—having a solute concentration greater than that of another solution.

Hypotonic—having a lesser solute concentration than that of another solution.

Isotonic—having the same solute concentration as that of another solution.

normal cell physiology requires that the concentration of potassium be higher within the cell than outside the cell, whereas the concentration of sodium is higher outside the cell than inside. A mechanism referred to as the sodium-potassium ion pump actively moves potassium into the cell and sodium out of the cell.

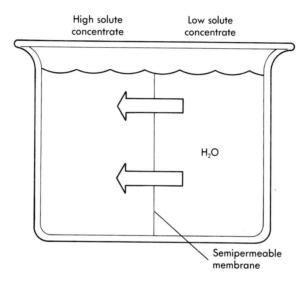

Figure 5-2 Movement of water by osmosis. (From Thelan LA, Davie JK, Urden LD: *Textbook of Critical Care Nursing*, St Louis, 1990, Mosby–Year Book.)

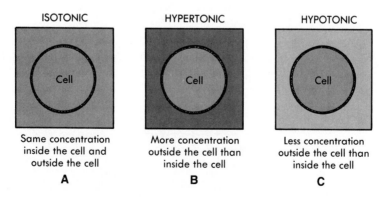

Figure 5-3 **A,** Isotonic solution. The extracellular solution concentration is the same as the intracellular concentration. There is no movement of water into or out of the cell. **B,** Hypertonic solution. The extracellular solution concentration is greater than the intracellular concentration. Water moves from the cell into the extracellular compartment. **C,** Hypotonic solution. The extracellular solution concentration is less than the intracellular concentration. Water moves from the extracellular compartment into the cell. (From Thelan LA, Davie JK, Urden LD: *Textbook of Critical Care Nursing*, St Louis, 1990, Mosby–Year Book.)

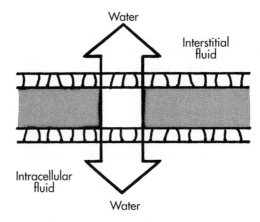

Figure 5-4   The effect of isotonic solutions on the movement of water across the cell membrane.

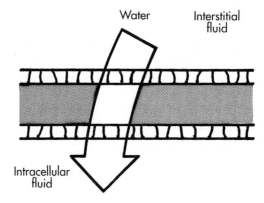

Figure 5-5   The effect of hypotonic solutions on the movement of water across the cell membrane.

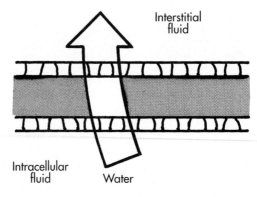

Figure 5-6   The effect of hypertonic solutions on the movement of water across the cell membrane.

IV FLUIDS

IV fluids, although not commonly considered drugs, are indeed drugs by definition. On-line medical direction or standing orders are required for the administration of IV fluids. The principles of drug administration discussed in Chapter 3 apply to all IV fluid therapy.

There are two major categories of IV fluids: **colloids** and **crystalloids.** Colloids contain compounds of high molecular weight, such as protein molecules, that do not readily cross the cell membrane. This causes the colloid solution to remain in the intravascular space for extended periods of time. In addition, the presence of the large molecules in colloids result in an osmotic pressure (referred to as **colloid osmotic pressure**) that is greater than the osmotic pressure of interstitial and intracellular fluid. This causes fluid to move from the interstitial and intracellular spaces into the intravascular space, resulting in increased intravascular volume. For this reason, colloids are often referred to as *volume expanders.*

Whole blood and blood products are examples of colloids. Because colloids are expensive and have short shelf lives, they are not usually carried by emergency medical service organizations. However, paramedics sometimes administer colloids during interhospital transfers.

Crystalloid solutions contain electrolytes and water. The dissolved ions contained in crystalloid solutions cross the cell membrane, and therefore remain in the intravascular space for only a short time before being distributed throughout the interstitial space. Crystalloid solutions, such as normal saline and lactated Ringer's, are commonly used in the prehospital setting

Another commonly used fluid in the prehospital setting is 5% dextrose in water (D_5W). D_5W contains dextrose and free water, which leave the intravascular space almost immediately and provide little intravascular volume expansion.

IV FLUID THERAPY

In healthy individuals homeostasis is maintained by balancing the intake and output of fluids and electrolytes. In the ill or injured individual, however, this balance is not as easily maintained, and excesses or deficits can occur. Because specific electrolyte imbalances generally require laboratory data for definitive diagnosis, they are not usually managed in the prehospital setting and are best treated in the hospital setting. Fluid therapy, however, is an important aspect of patient management in prehospital care.

It is important that paramedics be able to determine when IV fluids are indicated and what kind of fluid should be used in specific situations. The major indication for fluid therapy in the field is hypovolemia. Hypovolemia occurs with any clinical condition that causes the loss of water and solutes from the extracellular fluid compartment, such as hemorrhage, burns, prolonged vomiting, severe diarrhea, profuse sweating, or diabetic ketoacidosis. Hypovolemia is characterized by pale, clammy skin, weak peripheral pulses, increased heart rate, increased respiratory rate, decreased blood pressure, and reduced urinary output.

Isotonic crystalloids (normal saline or lactated Ringer's) are the fluids of choice for the treatment of hypovolemia in the prehospital setting. When isotonic crystalloids are administered, they are distributed between the interstitial and the intravascular compartments; little of the crystalloids enter the cell. After being infused, only about 20% of the crystalloid remains in the intravascular space, with the remaining volume (80%) moving into the interstitial space.[7] For this reason, 3 to 5 times the estimated volume lost must be administered.

Typically in adults, 100 to 500 ml are administered over 15 minutes to 1 hour. In severe hemorrhage, however, flow rates must be very high to accomplish adequate volume replacement, resulting in large quantities of crystalloid solution being administered over short periods of time. Achieving adequate infusion rates can present a challenge. The box below discusses methods of rapid infusion of fluids.

RAPID FLUID ADMINISTRATION

Administration of IV fluids in sufficient quantities to accomplish volume replacement in severe hypovolemia can be difficult. To accomplish this the American College of Surgeons Committee on Trauma recommends the initiation of two large-bore IV lines. Other methods that have been used to increase flow rates include: (1) use of a commercial pressure infuser (see photo); (2) manually squeezing the bag; (3) inflating a blood pressure cuff around the fluid bag; or (4) kneeling on the bag.

In a study conducted by White et al, it was demonstrated that applying a blood pressure cuff and kneeling on the IV bag were no more effective than gravity alone, and they recommended that use of these methods be discontinued.[9] Manually squeezing the bag was found to provide average flow rates 1.5 times greater than gravity alone. Use of a pressure infuser, capable of delivering 300 to 350 ml/min via standard IV tubing and a 14-gauge IV catheter, was found to be most effective. The researchers recommended that ambulances stock at least two pressure infusers and that medical directors mandate use of pressure infusers for patients in need of fluid resuscitation.[9]

In infants and children with hypovolemia, lactated Ringer's is the fluid of choice. Fluids are administered by bolus instead of at a steady rate as in adults. Crystalloids should be administered at 20 ml/kg as rapidly as possible, and the child reassessed. The bolus should be repeated as needed, based on continued reassessment of the child.[2]

A positive response to fluid therapy in children and adults is indicated by satisfactory mental status, normal heart rate, capillary refill of less than 2 seconds, and improved skin color. Paramedics must continually monitor the patient's response to fluid therapy and, in consultation with medical direction, adjust flow rates accordingly.

Administering large volumes of crystalloid solutions at rapid rates is not without side effects. Fluid overload is a common complication of aggressive fluid resuscitation.[3] (Signs and symptoms of fluid overload are presented in Chapter 3.) Rapid replacement with large quantities of crystalloids can also result in hypothermia, which has been identified as a poor prognostic indicator in severe trauma.[9]

Just as it is important that paramedics recognize the need for aggressive fluid replacement, it is equally important that paramedics know when fluids should be limited. Patients with congestive heart failure or pulmonary edema generally require IV access for the administration of medications. However, these patients tolerate fluids very poorly because of the inadequacy of their hearts' pumping action. IVs in such cases should be monitored judiciously, and just enough fluid should be administered to maintain IV access (usually less than 50 ml/hr). Patients who are at risk for developing increased intracranial pressure, such as those with head injuries, should also have restricted fluid intake.

D_5W is used frequently in the prehospital setting when large volumes of fluid are not needed. D_5W is isotonic in the container, but when administered, the dextrose molecules leave circulation so rapidly that its effect is that of a hypotonic solution. It is distributed in the intracellular compartment, hydrating the cell, and can cause significant edema.

D_5W is the fluid of choice for keep-open IVs and the administration of medications. D_5W is compatible with most medications; there are, however, a few exceptions, such as phenytoin. When giving phenytoin intravenously, normal saline should be used for the primary line. If D_5W is used, the tubing should be flushed with normal saline before and after giving phenytoin.

Lactated Ringer's, normal saline, and D_5W are the most commonly administered IV fluids in the prehospital setting. Ten percent dextrose ($D_{10}W$), 0.45% sodium chloride (half normal saline), and 5% dextrose in 0.45% sodium chloride are used less frequently. Table 5-2 summarizes the use of all these fluids in the prehospital setting.

Table 5-2 Commonly Used Crystalloids and Colloids

SOLUTION	DESCRIPTION	INDICATIONS	CONTRAINDICATIONS	RATE OF ADMINISTRATION	HOW SUPPLIED
Crystalloids					
Lactated Ringer's (Hartman's solution)	An isotonic crystalloid solution. One liter of lactated Ringer's contains 130 mEq of sodium (Na^+), 4 mEq of potassium (K^+), 3 mEq of calcium (Ca^{++}), 109 mEq of chlorine (Cl^-), and 28 mEq of lactate.	Hypovolemia	None in life-threatening hypovolemia	In hypovolemic shock, lactated Ringer's should be infused at a very rapid rate (wide open) until a systolic blood pressure of 100 mm Hg is achieved. Thereafter the rate should be **titrated** in response to the patient's blood pressure. With a stable blood pressure, a rate of 100 ml/hr is appropriate.	250, 500, and 1000 ml bags and bottles
0.9% Sodium chloride (normal saline)	An isotonic crystalloid solution. One liter of normal saline contains 154 mEq of sodium ions (Na^+) and 154 mEq of chloride ions (Cl^-)	Diabetic ketoacidosis Heat exhaustion Hypovolemia Keep-open IV*	None in life-threatening hypovolemia	The rate is determined by the patient's condition. In heat exhaustion or diabetic ketoacidosis it may be necessary to administer fluid rapidly. In other less emergent situations a moderate rate of administration (100 ml/hr) is appropriate.	250, 500, and 1000 ml (smaller volumes of 50 or 100 ml are available for mixing medications)
0.45% Sodium chloride (half normal saline)	A hypotonic solution. Contains half the concentration of NaCl as blood plasma.	Patients with decreased renal or cardiac function	Should not be used for volume replacement in hypovolemia	The rate is determined by the patient's condition.\	250, 500, 1000 ml bags and bottles
5% Dextrose in water	A hypotonic solution	Keep-open IV Dilution of drugs for administration	Pulmonary edema Cerebral edema Renal failure Should not be used for volume replacement in hypovolemia	The rate at which D_5W is administered is determined by the specific circumstances. Often in the prehospital setting D_5W is administered at a keep-open rate.	50, 100, 150, 250, 500, and 1000 ml bags (the smaller volumes are usually used for diluting medications prior to administration)

5% Dextrose in 0.45% sodium chloride	Contains dextrose (80 calories/L) and half normal saline.	Heat exhaustion Diabetes Keep-open IV for patients with impaired renal or cardiac function	Should not be used for volume replacement in hypovolemia	The rate is determined by the patient's condition.	250, 500, and 1000 ml bags and bottles
10% Dextrose (D$_{10}$W)	A hypertonic solution. Used when volume replacement is not indicated. Its carbohydrate content makes it useful in hypoglycemia.	Hypoglycemia Neonatal resuscitation	Should not be used for volume replacement in hypovolemia	The rate is determined by the patient's condition.	50, 100, 150, 250, 500, and 1000 ml bags
Colloids					
Plasma protein fraction (Plasmanate)	Serum human albumin (plasma protein) suspended in saline solvent.	Hypovolemic shock (especially burn shock)	None in life-threatening hypovolemia	The rate is titrated to the patient's physiologic response.	250 and 500 ml bottles of 5% solution
Dextran	Contains chains of sugars that are nearly the same molecular weight as serum albumin	Hypovolemic shock	Hypersensitivity	The rate is titrated to the patient's physiologic response	Available as dextran 40 and dextran 70 in 250 and 500 ml bottles
Hetastarch (Hespan)	An artificial colloid derived from amylopectin (chemically similar to glycogen)	Hypovolemic shock	None in life-threatening hypovolemia	The rate is titrated to the patient's physiologic response.	500 ml bottles of 6% hetastarch in 0.9% NaCl

*Normal saline is sometimes used for keep-open IVs. When used as a keep-open IV for patients with congestive heart failure, the rate must be regulated carefully and the patient observed closely for fluid overload.

SUMMARY

Fluid and electrolyte balance is essential to life. The safe and timely administration of the appropriate IV fluid is an important aspect of prehospital care. The fluids most often used in the prehospital setting are lactated Ringer's, normal saline, and D_5W. Lactated Ringer's and normal saline are used primarily in hypovolemic patients. D_5W is generally used to establish IV access and maintained as a keep-open IV.

REFERENCES

1. Beck RK: *Pharmacology for prehospital emergency care*, 76, Philadelphia, 1992, FA Davis.
2. Chameides L, editor: *Textbook of pediatric advanced life support*, 24, 1988, American Heart Association.
3. Griffel MI, Kaufman BS: Pharmacology of colloids and crystalloids, *Crit Care Clin* 8(2):235, 1992.
4. Keweski SM, Suise MJ, Virgilio RW: The effects of prehospital fluids on survival in trauma patients, *J Trauma* 30:1215, 1990.
5. Porth CM: *Pathophysiology: concepts of altered health states*, ed 3, Philadelphia, 1990, JB Lippincott.
6. Rottman SJ, Larmon B, Manix T: Rapid volume infusion in prehospital care, *Prehosp Disast Med* 5(3):225.
7. Sommers M: Rapid fluid resuscitation—how to correct dangerous deficits, *Nursing 90* 20(1):52, 1990.
8. Thelan LA, Davie JK, Urden LD: *Textbook of critical care nursing-diagnosis and management*, St. Louis, 1990, Mosby–Year Book.
9. White SJ, Hamilton WA, Veronesi JF: A comparison of field techniques used to pressure-infuse intravenous fluids, *Prehosp Disast Med* 6(2):129, 1991.

6
The Autonomic Nervous System

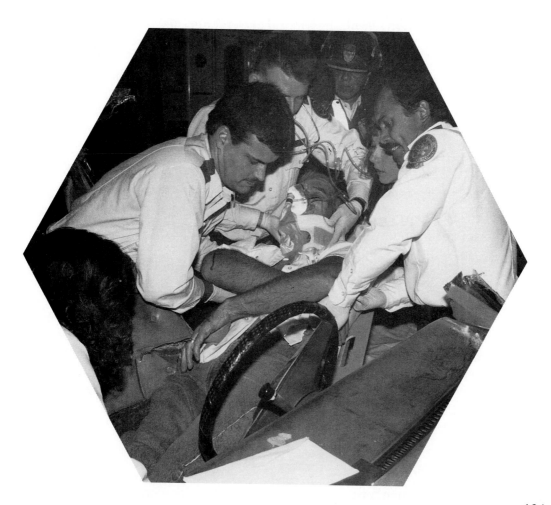

OBJECTIVES

1. Describe the functions of the sympathetic and parasympathetic nervous systems.
2. Explain how the sympathetic nervous system supports the body's response to stress.
3. Explain how autonomic nerve impulses are transmitted.
4. Define cholinergic and adrenergic receptors.
5. Discuss the effects of alpha adrenergic and beta adrenergic stimulation on vital organs.
6. Describe the mechanisms by which autonomic drugs exert their actions.

The autonomic nervous system is the part of the peripheral nervous system that regulates involuntary body functions. It controls such vital functions as the body's response to stress, cardiac rhythm, blood pressure, and blood flow to the brain, heart, and skeletal muscles.

Many drugs administered in the prehospital setting act by stimulating or blocking autonomic responses. Understanding the autonomic nervous system is essential to understanding drug therapy. This chapter discusses the major divisions of the autonomic nervous system, the transmission of autonomic impulses, and the various autonomic receptors that drugs act on.

STRUCTURE AND FUNCTION OF THE AUTONOMIC NERVOUS SYSTEM

The autonomic nervous system is structurally and functionally divided into two parts: the sympathetic nervous system and the parasympathetic nervous system. Many organs are innervated by both sympathetic and parasympathetic fibers that are continually active at a baseline level (basal rate). The effect of this constant stimulation is referred to as "tone."

Generally, an organ is predominantly controlled by either the sympathetic or parasympathetic system. The tone of a specific organ can be increased or decreased by changes in the level of stimulation of the predominant system. For example, the sinoatrial and atrioventricular nodes are innervated by both sympathetic and parasympathetic fibers, but the parasympathetic system dominates. During times of normal activity the parasympathetic nervous system controls heart rate by exerting an inhibitory effect via the vagus nerve. During times of physical or emotional stress the sympathetic nervous system overrides parasympathetic tone and heart rate increases.

Sympathetic Nervous System

The sympathetic nervous system is primarily concerned with the regulation of temperature, cardiovascular function, and the body's response to stress. The sympathetic nervous system regulates body temperature by controlling blood flow to the skin and stimulating perspiration.

Cardiovascular function is influenced by the sympathetic nervous system's effect on heart rate, contractility, conduction velocity, and vascular smooth muscle. Sympathetic stimulation increases heart rate, force of cardiac contraction, and conduction velocities, thereby increasing cardiac output. It also influences blood pressure and tissue perfusion by constricting vascular smooth muscle (vasoconstriction).

The sympathetic nervous system plays an important role in emergencies. An understanding of the generalized and widespread response of the sympathetic nervous system in times of stress is important. When faced with danger, the body's physiologic response is to prepare to fight or flee. This is referred to as the *fight or flight response* (Figure 6-1). The sympathetic nervous system increases the firing frequency of sympathetic fibers and activates sympathetic fibers that are normally silent. This results in: (1) shunting of blood from the periphery and viscera to skeletal muscle; (2) increased cardiac output; (3) increased blood sugar; and (4) dilation of the pupils.

Parasympathetic Nervous System

Generally, the parasympathetic nervous system is associated with promoting the conservation of energy and maintaining vital functions during periods of rest. It has been described as being concerned with the "housekeeping" or "vegetative" functions of the body. Specific regulatory functions of the parasympathetic nervous system include focusing the eye for near vision, constricting the pupils, emptying the bowels and urinary bladder, increasing gastric secretion, and slowing the heart rate.

Transmission of Impulses

In both systems nerve impulses are transmitted through **preganglionic fibers (axons)**, **ganglia**, and **postganglionic axons**. Preganglionic axons conduct impulses from the spinal cord to the ganglia. From the ganglia, postganglionic axons conduct impulses to the **effector organ**.

KEY TERMS

Ganglia—a mass of nerve cells.

Effector organ—an organ or group of tissues on which the autonomic nervous system exerts an effect; target organ.

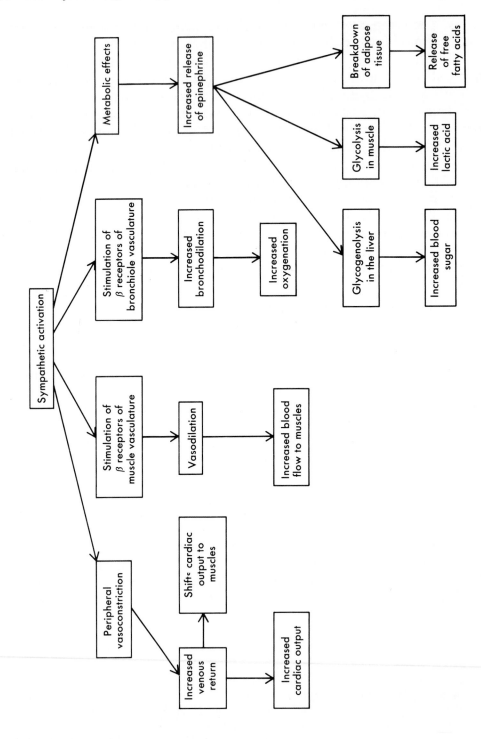

Figure 6-1   Fight or flight response. (From McCance KL, Huether SE: *Pathophysiology: the biologic basis for disease in adults and children*, St Louis, 1990, Mosby–Year Book.)

The junction between the axon and the ganglia or the effector organ is referred to as a **synapse**. For transmission of nerve impulses to occur, chemical substances called **neurotransmitters** must be present at the synapse. **Norepinephrine** and **acetylcholine** are the primary neurotransmitters in the autonomic nervous system. Acetylcholine is released by preganglionic fibers in both the sympathetic and parasympathetic nervous systems and by the postganglionic fibers in the parasympathetic nervous system. These impulses are referred to as **cholinergic**. Norepinephrine is released by the postganglionic fibers of the sympathetic nervous system. These impulses are referred to as **adrenergic**. (Note: in the sweat glands the postganglionic fibers release acetylcholine.) Figure 6-2 illustrates the parasympathetic and sympathetic transmission of impulses.

Endocrine hormones can also act as neurotransmitters. As part of the physiologic response to stress the autonomic nervous system stimulates the **adrenal medulla,** which in turn secretes norepinephrine and epinephrine. These hormones are chemically similar to each other and have adrenergic effects.

Receptors

Understanding receptors is fundamental to understanding the actions of autonomic drugs. Knowing the receptors at which a specific drug acts and the response usually mediated by that receptor, one can predict the effects of a drug.

Cholinergic receptors. Cholinergic receptors are those that respond to the neurotransmitter acetylcholine. Table 6-1 summarizes the body's response to cholinergic and adrenergic stimulation. Drugs that elicit a response similar to acetylcholine are referred to as cholinergic or parasympathomimetic. Drugs that block cholinergic responses are referred to as anticholinergic or parasympatholytic. There are two types of cholinergic receptors: nicotinic and muscarinic. Nicotinic receptors are located in all autonomic ganglia, the adrenal medulla, and striated muscle. Muscarinic receptors are found in the heart, smooth muscle, and glands. Atropine sulfate, a drug used frequently in the prehospital setting, is an example of an antimuscarinic (anticholinergic) agent.

KEY TERM

Adrenal medulla—a secretory organ located on top of the kidney that manufactures and secretes epinephrine and norepinephrine.

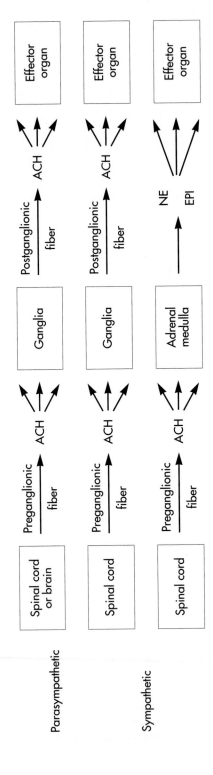

Figure 6-2   Transmission of impulses in the autonomic nervous system.

Adrenergic receptors. Adrenergic receptors are those receptors that respond to the neurotransmitters norepinephrine and epinephrine. Dopamine, a precursor in the formation of epinephrine, can also act as a neurotransmitter in the sympathetic nervous system. Drugs that mediate an adrenergic response are referred to as adrenergic or sympathomimetic. Drugs that block or inhibit adrenergic receptors are called antiadrenergic or sympatholytic. There are four types of adrenergic receptors: alpha$_1$, alpha$_2$, beta$_1$, and beta$_2$. The effects of stimulating each of these receptors are shown in Table 6-1.

Table 6-1 Actions of Autonomic Nerve Impulses on Specific Tissues

TISSUE	RECEPTOR SITE	ADRENERGIC RECEPTORS (SYMPATHETIC)	CHOLINERGIC RECEPTORS (PARASYMPATHETIC)
Blood vessels			
Arterioles			
Coronary	α; $\beta 2$	Constriction; dilation	Dilation
Skin	α	Constriction	Dilation
Renal	$\alpha 1$; $\beta 1$ & $\beta 2$	Constriction; dilation	—
Skeletal muscle	α; $\beta 2$	Constriction; dilation	Dilation
Veins (systemic)	$\alpha 1$; $\beta 2$	Constriction; dilation	—
Eye			
Radial muscle, iris	$\alpha 1$	Contraction (mydriasis)	—
Sphincter muscle, iris	—	—	Contraction (miosis)
Ciliary muscle	β	Relaxation for far vision	Contraction for near vision
Gastrointestinal tract			
Smooth muscle	α; $\beta 1$ & $\beta 2$	Relaxation	Contraction
Sphincters	α	Contraction	Relaxation
Heart	$\beta 1$	Increased heartrate	Decreased heartrate
Lung			
Bronchial muscle	$\beta 2$	Smooth muscle relaxation (opens airways)	Smooth muscle contraction (closes airways)
Bronchial glands	$\alpha 1$; $\beta 2$	Decreased secretions; increased secretions	Stimulation
Urinary bladder			
Fundus (detrusor)	β	Relaxation	Contraction
Trigone and sphincter	α	Contraction	Relaxation
Uterus	α; $\beta 2$	Pregnant: contraction (α); relaxation (β_2)	Variable

From Clayton BD, Stock YN: *Basic pharmacology for nurses*, ed 10, St Louis, 1993, Mosby–Year Book.
*α, Alpha receptors; β_1, Beta 1 receptors; β_2, Beta 2 receptors.

Alpha₁ receptors are located in the eyes, reproductive organs, and blood vessels. The alpha₁ receptors of the eyes and reproductive organs have less relevance in emergency medicine than those of the blood vessels. Stimulation of the alpha₁ receptors results in the contraction of vascular smooth muscle and, therefore, vasoconstriction. Some of the drugs that are used to raise arterial blood pressure do so by stimulating alpha receptors.

Alpha₂ receptors regulate transmitter release and are of little significance in autonomic drugs. Alpha₂ receptors in the central nervous system are relevant to the treatment of hypertension.

Beta₁ receptors are located in the heart and kidneys. Stimulation of the beta₁ receptors results in increased heart rate, increased force of contraction, and increased conduction velocity in the His-Purkinje system of the heart. Stimulation of the beta₁ receptors in the kidneys results in the release of renin, which ultimately elevates blood pressure.

Beta₂ receptors are located in the eyes, salivary glands, bronchioles, stomach, liver, pancreas, intestines, skin, skeletal muscle, lungs, and arterioles of the heart. Stimulation of the beta₂ receptors of the bronchioles causes bronchodilation. Many of the drugs used in respiratory emergencies are given for their ability to stimulate beta₂ receptors. Stimulation of the beta receptors in the arterioles of the heart, lungs, and skeletal muscle causes vasodilation, resulting in increased perfusion to these organs.

AUTONOMIC DRUGS

Drugs that exert their effect within the autonomic nervous system act either on specific receptor sites or along the transmission pathway. Autonomic drugs generally affect the entire body rather than specific organs. The effects of autonomic drugs depends on which part of the autonomic nervous system they interact with and whether they stimulate or inhibit that system. There are many synonymous terms used to describe drugs that act on the autonomic nervous system. Table 6-2 clarifies these terms.

Sympathetic Drugs

Adrenergic (sympathomimetic) drugs are commonly used in the prehospital setting, particularly within the Advanced Cardiac Life Support algorithms. These drugs are indicated mainly for their effect on the heart, blood vessels, and bronchi. Because of the number and location of adrenergic receptors in the body, adrenergic drugs have a profound systemic effect. Depending on the dose, the reason for use, and the route of administration,

Table 6-2 Common Synonyms for Autonomic Terminology

TERM	SYNONYM
adrenergic	sympathetic sympathomimetic alpha adrenergic beta adrenergic
antiadrenergic	sympatholytic adrenergic blocker sympathetic blocker alpha blocker beta blocker
cholinergic	parasympathetic parasympathomimetic
anticholinergic	parasympatholytic cholinergic blocker parasympathetic blocker

an adrenergic drug can have both therapeutic and adverse effects. For example, when epinephrine is administered in a respiratory emergency for its bronchodilating effect, it can also increase an already elevated heart rate. It is important to recognize what effects an adrenergic drug will have, in addition to the desired effect for which it is being administered.

Antiadrenergic (sympatholytic) agents block adrenergic receptors of the sympathetic nervous system. Antiadrenergic drugs are most commonly used in the long-term treatment of hypertension. Adrenergic blocking agents can either be alpha-adrenergic blockers or beta-adrenergic blockers. Alpha-adrenergic blocking agents have limited use. Beta-adrenergic blocking agents are indicated in the treatment of dysrhythmias, hypertension, angina pectoris, and myocardial infarction. Beta-blockers are used infrequently in the prehospital setting and generally limited to those with antidysrhythmic properties, such as propranolol.

Parasympathetic Drugs

Cholinergic (parasympathomimetic) drugs are drugs that stimulate cholinergic receptors. These drugs are used primarily in the treatment of glaucoma and neuromuscular disease and, therefore, have little application in prehospital care.

Anticholinergic drugs block the effects of acetylcholine on cholinergic receptors. Atropine sulfate is a commonly used anticholinergic drug.

Atropine is used in the field for symptomatic bradycardias and organophosphate poisoning.

Parasympathetic stimulation causes a decrease in heart rate via its action on the vagus nerve. Atropine blocks parasympathetic stimulation, thereby decreasing vagal tone and increasing heart rate. In organophosphate poisoning there is a generalized overstimulation of the parasympathetic nervous system. Atropine is typically given in large doses to block these effects.

SUMMARY

The autonomic nervous system is responsible for maintaining a constant internal environment. It is divided into two major parts: sympathetic and parasympathetic. The autonomic nervous system is vital to the maintenance of blood pressure, respiratory status, and cardiac rhythm. Drugs that affect the autonomic nervous system are commonly used in emergency intervention. In the remaining chapters these drugs are profiled where appropriate.

REFERENCES

1. Clayton BD: *Basic pharmacology for nurses*, ed 10, St Louis, 1993, Mosby–Year Book.
2. Collins AC: *Clinical drug therapy*, ed 2, Philadelphia, 1987, JB Lippincott.
3. McCance KL, Huether SE: *Pathophysiology: the biologic basis for disease in adults and children*, St Louis, 1990, Mosby–Year Book.
4. Porth CM: *Pathophysiology—concepts of altered health states*, ed 3, Philadelphia, 1990, JB Lippincott.
5. American Heart Association: *Textbook of advanced cardiac life support*, ed 2, 1987, American Heart Association.

7
Respiratory Emergencies

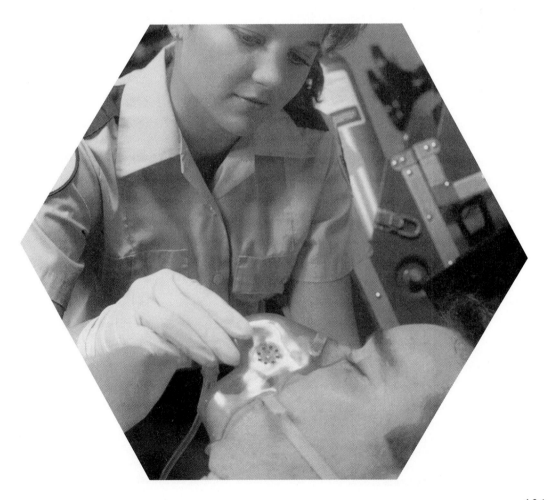

OBJECTIVES

1. List factors that influence tissue oxygenation.
2. Discuss the management of hypoxia in the prehospital setting.
3. Differentiate among methods of oxygen administration.
4. Define obstructive airway disease.
5. Discuss the pharmacologic management of obstructive airway disease in the prehospital setting.
6. Discuss the use of epinephrine in acute bronchospasm.
7. Describe the advantages of the beta$_2$ agonists in the treatment of acute bronchospasm.
8. Discuss the advantages of administering beta$_2$ agonists via inhalation.
9. Explain the role of corticosteroids in the treatment of acute asthma.
10. Discuss the pharmacologic management of respiratory distress associated with anaphylaxis.
11. Relate indications, mechanisms of action, side effects, and administration precautions for selected pharmacologic agents.

Respiratory emergencies vary widely in etiology and complexity. Providing adequate tissue oxygenation is a fundamental concern for all patients. This chapter addresses the principles of tissue oxygenation and the administration of oxygen, focusing on the various methods of oxygen delivery.

DRUGS PROFILED IN THIS CHAPTER

CLASSIFICATION	DRUG	PAGE
Antihistamine	Diphenhydramine hydrochloride	154
Anticholinergic	Ipratropium bromide	155
Corticosteroid	Methylprednisolone	156
Gas	Oxygen	157
Sympathomimetic bronchodilator	Albuterol sulfate	152
	Terbutaline sulfate	159
Xanthine derivative	Aminophylline	153

The pharmacologic management of respiratory emergencies related to obstructive airway disease (e.g., asthma, bronchitis, and emphysema) and anaphylaxis are also presented. The major drug groups discussed in this chapter are sympathomimetic bronchodilators, xanthine derivatives, corticosteroids, antihistamines, and anticholinergics.

◆ CASE PRESENTATIONS

Case Presentation 1 (Pneumonia)

At 4:15 PM, paramedics respond to a call and find a 53-year-old, 55-kg female complaining of shortness of breath. She is awake, restless, and sitting up in bed. She appears to be in moderate distress with labored breathing. History reveals fever and chills for the past 24 hours, complaints of sharp pain on the right side of the chest, nausea, and vomiting. She denies any history of chronic obstructive pulmonary disease and is not taking any medications at this time.

The physical exam reveals: P-122, R-30, BP-110/86, skin warm to touch, crackles in all right lung fields. The paramedics apply a pulse oximeter and place her on a cardiac monitor. The pulse oximeter indicates that her oxygen saturation is 78%, and the cardiac monitor shows sinus tachycardia.

The patient is given oxygen via a simple face mask at 8 L/min and transported to the nearest hospital. After 5 minutes of oxygen therapy, a second set of vital signs reveals a change in pulse rate from 122 to 100, a reduction of respiratory rate from 30 to 26, and an increase in oxygen saturation to 90%. Subsequent evaluation in the emergency department confirms a diagnosis of pneumonia.

Case Presentation 2 (Asthma)

Paramedics respond to the home of a 13-year-old, 45 kg male who reportedly became increasingly short of breath over the past hour. The patient's history reveals he is taking Theo-Dur orally and using a Ventolin inhaler. He has had upper respiratory infection symptoms and a persistent cough for 2 days. He is now severely short of breath. He is awake and alert, although only able to speak one word at a time. He has retractions and is using all accessory muscles.

Vital signs are: P-140, R-40, BP-136/82. His skin is warm and dry. Diffuse inspiratory and expiratory wheezes are heard in all lung fields. After initiating oxygen at 3 L/min via nasal cannula and administering albuterol by hand-held nebulizer, the patient's shortness of breath improves. ◆

TISSUE OXYGENATION

Tissue oxygenation depends on several factors: adequate **ventilation**, the concentration of oxygen in inhaled air, gas exchange across the alveoli, and blood flow for oxygen transport to the tissues. Changes in any one of these factors can result in **hypoxia**. Signs and symptoms of tissue hypoxia include restlessness, anxiety, tachycardia, tachypnea, dysrhythmias, cyanosis, and drowsiness.

The causes of hypoxia are divided into four categories: (1) hypoxemia, an insufficient amount of oxygen in arterial blood; (2) ischemic or stagnant hypoxia, in which there is inadequate circulation to the tissues, as seen in shock; (3) anemic hypoxia, in which oxygen transport in the blood is

---

PULSE OXIMETRY

Pulse oximetry is a noninvasive method of measuring oxygen saturation that is being used with increasing frequency in the prehospital setting. Simply stated, the pulse oximeter works by analyzing the absorption of red and infrared light in arterial blood via a small sensor applied to an arterial bed, usually the finger or earlobe. It provides an immediate and continuous reading of oxygen saturation and pulse rate. Data is displayed in a digital or graphic form.

Oxygen saturation is a good indicator of respiratory status. Oxygen saturation should be greater than 90%. Values less than 90% are indicative of hypoxemia. Pulse oximetry provides for the prompt recognition of hypoxemia and enables paramedics to assess the efficacy of airway management and oxygen therapy.

KEY TERM

Hypoxia—inadequate tissue oxygenation; reduced tension of cellular oxygen.

decreased, as seen with decreased hemoglobin levels; and (4) histotoxic hypoxia, in which the cells are unable to use oxygen, as seen with some poisonings (e.g., cyanide).

Tissue hypoxia can occur with many types of respiratory emergencies, including pneumonia, acute asthma, pulmonary edema, airway obstruction, smoke inhalation, and bronchospasm. Nonrespiratory emergencies that can lead to tissue hypoxia include hemorrhage, shock, and cardiac events, such as myocardial infarction and congestive heart failure.

The overall status of tissue oxygenation is reflected in the oxygen saturation of hemoglobin. Pulse oximeters provide paramedics with a quick and accurate means of objectively measuring oxygen saturation and, if available, should be used for all patients at risk for developing hypoxia (see box on page 134).

PREHOSPITAL MANAGEMENT OF HYPOXIA

The primary intervention for hypoxia is the administration of oxygen. Because oxygen is the most commonly administered drug in the prehospital setting, its benefits are often taken for granted. The importance of oxygen therapy in the field cannot be overstated.

Both case presentations in this chapter illustrate the importance of oxygen administration for patients with hypoxia. In Case Presentation 1 the patient's initial presentation and history suggested pneumonia. However, a definitive diagnosis was not possible nor is it necessary in the field. The critical issue for this patient was her shortness of breath and the accompanying changes in vital signs. It is clear that the patient was hypoxic: restlessness, tachycardia, tachypnea, shortness of breath, and crackles are all signs. Regardless of etiology, the priority in patient management is to improve tissue oxygenation. Similarly, the patient in Case Presentation 2 appeared to have significant hypoxia, evidenced by his increased respiratory rate, use of accessory muscles, and wheezing. His history and symptoms suggested asthma, but the critical issue is hypoxia. He required the immediate administration of oxygen.

OXYGEN ADMINISTRATION

Oxygen administration provides patients with a higher concentration of oxygen than is normally present in atmospheric air. This increased concentration of oxygen is delivered to the alveoli, which in turn increases the amount of oxygen in the blood available for transport to the tissues.

Oxygen should be administered in any situation in which tissue hypoxia is likely to occur. (See drug profile at the end of this chapter for specific indications.) Generally, adults, infants, and children who demonstrate signs and symptoms of acute respiratory distress should be given oxygen at the highest concentration available. In emergencies in which respiratory distress is not apparent but the underlying pathology may lead to hypoxia (e.g., myocardial infarction and multiple trauma), supplemental oxygen should be administered.

Oxygen should be used cautiously in patients who are known to have chronic obstructive pulmonary disease (COPD). Normally, the stimulus for respiration is a rise in the level of carbon dioxide (CO_2) in the blood. Patients with COPD may have chronic carbon dioxide retention, resulting in decreased responsiveness to changes in carbon dioxide levels. Their stimulus for respiration is dependent then on peripheral chemoreceptors sensing low oxygen levels (hypoxemia). This is referred to as *hypoxic drive*. There is the potential in such circumstances for patients to respond to oxygen administration with a rise in carbon dioxide level and periods of apnea. This presents the paramedics with a real dilemma. Research suggests that fear of inducing central nervous system depression (which occurs with elevated carbon dioxide levels) has caused some providers to be overcautious in administering oxygen.[15]

In cases of severe respiratory distress the correction of hypoxemia is crucial. Severe hypoxia can lead to irreversible brain damage in minutes, whereas the changes seen with increased levels of carbon dioxide are reversible. *Therefore oxygen should never be withheld from a hypoxic patient for any reason.* Oxygen should be administered at low flow rates and the patient monitored for changes in level of consciousness and respiratory effort. Paramedics should be prepared to manage the airway via bag-valve mask or endotracheal intubation if necessary.

Methods of Oxygen Administration

For use in the field, oxygen is supplied in steel or aluminum cylinders. These cylinders are color-coded according to their contents. In the United States oxygen cylinders are green, as are all necessary regulators (reducing valves). Regulators control the flow of gas from a cylinder by reducing the high pressure in the cylinder to a safer range (50 psi) as the gas flows out. Because oxygen is stored under such high pressure, it can be dangerous if not handled properly (see box on page 137 for safety precautions).

To administer oxygen from a cylinder the following steps should be followed:

1. Using the supplied wrench, slowly and slightly open the cylinder valve

---

SAFETY PRECAUTIONS IN HANDLING OXYGEN CYLINDERS

- Cylinders should be secured at all times to prevent jarring or falling.
- Cylinders should not be subjected to extreme heat (temperatures above 125°F).
- Never attempt to open an oxygen cylinder without a properly fitting regulator valve in place. Regulator valves should be designated for use with oxygen only.
- When the oxygen cylinder is not in use, all valves should be closed.
- When working with oxygen cylinders, paramedics should always be positioned to the side of the cylinder out of the path of flow. In the event that the regulator is blown off, serious injury and even death can result.
- Oxygen cylinders and equipment should be inspected daily.
- All combustible materials should be kept clear of oxygen cylinders (e.g., oil, gas, and smoking materials). Smoking should not be permitted anywhere near oxygen cylinders.

---

and then quickly close it. This cracks the cylinder, preparing it for use, and clears the cylinder valve of any collected debris.

2. Inspect the regulator valve to ensure it is to be used with oxygen only. Apply the regulator valve and tighten securely.
3. Pressurize the regulator valve by slowly opening the cylinder valve. A needle or ball in the regulator valve indicates pressurization.
4. Apply the humidification source and delivery device.
5. Open the control valve on the regulator to desired flow.
6. After use, first shut off the control valve on the regulator, then shut off the main cylinder valve.
7. Open the control valve again to bleed the system, then close it when the indicator returns to zero.

Oxygen is administered by inhalation. Several methods of delivery are available, each with advantages and disadvantages (see Table 7-1). The specific method used for administration is determined by the condition of the patient and the concentration of oxygen desired. Regardless of the method of administration, unhumidified oxygen can cause drying of secretions and irritation of the mucous membranes. Some emergency medical services (EMS) systems do not use humidifiers when transport times are short. However, if transport time exceeds 15 to 20 minutes, a humidifier should be used. A humidifier consists simply of a jar of water and a flow meter. Most EMS systems today use disposable humidifiers. Humidification is particularly important in infants and young children because dried secretions can obstruct their small airways.

Oxygen administration systems can be divided into *low-flow* and *high-flow* systems. A high-flow system ejects the gas at such a rate that the amount of air provided is adequate to meet all the patient's inspiratory vol-

Table 7-1 Oxygen Delivery Methods

METHOD	FLOW RATE USED	% OXYGEN DELIVERED	COMMENTS
Nasal cannula	1-6	24-44	Comfortable, generally well-tolerated
Transtracheal catheter	2-4	50-60	Limited use in the field
Simple face mask	6-10	30-60	Usually well-tolerated in short-term therapy
Partial rebreathing mask	10-12	50-60	Usually well-tolerated in short-term therapy
Nonrebreathing mask	10-12	90-100	Delivers highest O_2 concentration
Venturi mask	4	24	Limited use in the field. Generally used in long-term maintenance of COPD patients.
	4	28	
	8	35	
	8	40	

COPD, chronic obstructive pulmonary disease.

ume requirements (**tidal volume**). Examples of high-flow systems are nonbreathing masks and venturi masks.

Low-flow systems do not deliver enough volume to meet all ventilation requirements. Their efficiency is dependent on the patient's respiratory pattern and to what extent the patient's tidal volume becomes diluted with room air. Examples of low-flow systems are nasal cannula (prongs), partial rebreathing masks, simple face masks, and transtracheal catheters (see Table 7-1).

The nasal cannula (Figure 7-1, *A*) is the most common device used for delivering oxygen. It is well-tolerated by most patients because it is less restrictive than the face mask. Disadvantages are: (1) the oxygen concentration delivered varies with the patient's respiratory pattern, (2) the cannula can dry membranes, resulting in irritation and nasal congestion, and (3) it can cause soreness around the nostrils. The nasal cannula provides a 24%- to 44%-oxygen concentration. The flow rate should be set at 1 to 6 L/min. Flow rates any greater than 6 L/min will not increase the oxygen concentration delivered and can, in fact, further contribute to mucosal drying and irritation.

The simple face mask is a soft plastic disposable mask that can deliver an oxygen concentration of 30% to 60%, with a flow rate of 6 to 10 L/min. Oxygen concentration delivered is dependent on the patient's respiratory pattern and tidal volume. The mask is constructed with small holes on either side (Figure 7-1, *B*). Room air is drawn in during inspiration and mixes with the oxygen. Expired air exits via the same holes. Patients frequently complain of discomfort when using this mask because the mask tends to become sticky and hot.

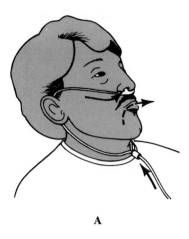

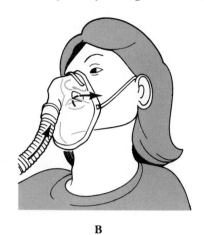

A

B

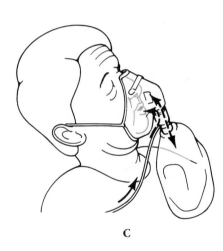

Figure 7-1 Various oxygen delivery systems. **A**, Nasal cannula. **B**, Simple face mask. **C**, Partial rebreathing mask. **D**, Nonrebreathing mask. **E**, Venturi mask. (From McKenry LM, Salerno E: Mosby's pharmacology in nursing, ed 18, St Louis, 1992, Mosby–Year Book.)

C

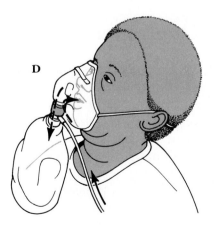

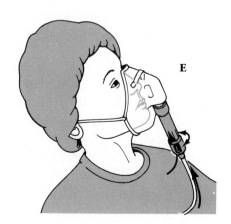

D

E

The transtracheal catheter is a fairly new method of oxygen delivery. The transtracheal catheter is surgically inserted directly into the trachea between the second and third tracheal cartilages. (This is not to be confused with transtracheal jet insufflation, an emergency ventilation technique used infrequently in the field when airway access with other methods is unobtainable.) The transtracheal catheter is generally used at home by patients who require continuous low-flow oxygen delivery, such as those with COPD. It is advantageous because it does not interfere with eating, drinking, or speaking, and it provides oxygen throughout the respiratory cycle, rather than only during inspiration. Although this method of delivery is not used in the field as a primary method of oxygen delivery, it may be encountered when responding to emergencies and in transport situations. When dealing with patients who have transtracheal catheters, great care should be taken to maintain the integrity of the system.

The partial rebreathing mask is a soft plastic, disposable mask attached to a reservoir bag and a partial rebreathing valve (Figure 7-1, C). When the patient exhales, approximately the first one-third of the expired air enters the reservoir and mixes with oxygen. This expired air is actually air that was in the patient's **dead space.** Gas exchange does not occur in this portion of the airway, so the exhaled air is oxygen enriched. The patient inspires a mix of the expired air and supplemental oxygen, allowing concentrations of 50% to 60% to be delivered using flow rates of 10 to 12 L/min.[3]

The nonrebreathing mask (Figure 7-1, D) resembles the partial rebreather in appearance because it also has a reservoir bag and a valve. Functionally, though, it is quite different because the one-way valve prevents expired air from mixing with the oxygen in the reservoir. All expired air exits out of the system via exhalation ports. The patient then inhales only oxygen from the reservoir bag. If a tight seal can be obtained with the mask, an oxygen concentration of 90% to 100% can be achieved with a flow rate of 10 to 12 L/min.[3] The major disadvantage of the nonrebreathing mask is the discomfort many patients experience. It becomes very hot and sticky, and most patients are unable to tolerate it for more than a few hours.

Like the transtracheal catheter, the Venturi mask is another system with limited use in the field (Figure 7-1, E). Paramedics will, however, encounter its use and perhaps be responsible for maintenance of the system during interhospital transports. The Venturi mask is designed to accurately provide predetermined concentrations of oxygen (24%, 28%, 35%, and 40%). This system is of particular value in patients with COPD who poorly tolerate high concentrations of oxygen.

All the systems described above are used with patients who have spontaneous respiratory effort. For nonbreathing patients, a bag-valve device is used along with a mask and oral airway, an endotracheal tube, or an esophageal obturator airway (Figure 7-2). The bag component is manually compressed to deliver ventilation. Bag-valve systems are designed much like the nonrebreathing mask system in that they have a nonrebreathing valve. When used with an oxygen flow of 10 to 12 L/min, it delivers 40% oxygen concentration. A reservoir bag may be added to the system, which increases the delivered oxygen concentration to 90% to 100%.

Agents other than oxygen may be used to facilitate tissue oxygenation. Any drug or IV fluid that acts to increase the blood pressure and/or to improve cardiac output indirectly increases oxygenation. These drugs are discussed in other chapters under specific systems. Drugs used to treat respiratory emergencies can be divided into three basic categories: (1) those used to increase the concentration of oxygen in inspired air (e.g., oxygen), (2) those that dilate the bronchioles (e.g., bronchodilators), and

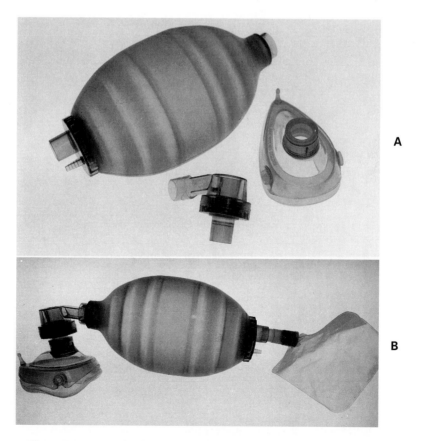

Figure 7-2 Bag-valve device. **A,** Without reservoir. **B,** With reservoir.

(3) those that interfere with chemical mediators (e.g., epinephrine, antihistamines, and corticosteroids).

OBSTRUCTIVE AIRWAY DISEASE

Asthma, bronchitis, and emphysema are referred to as obstructive airway diseases. Asthma and bronchitis cause reversible airway obstruction,

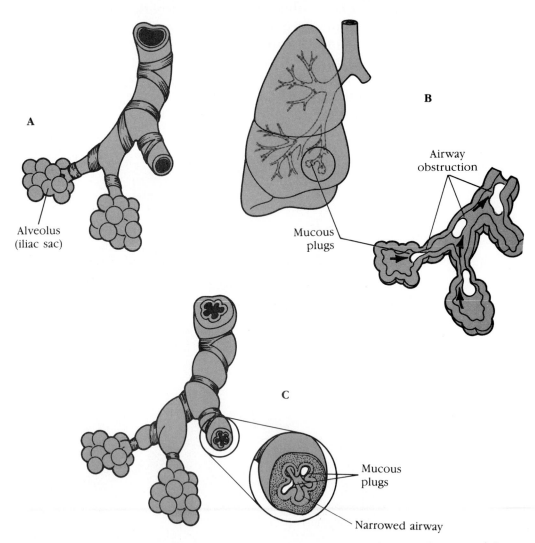

Figure 7-3 Bronchiole in **A,** normal state and **B,** during an asthma attack. **C,** Total amount of air inhaled and exhaled is decreased because of air trapped in the lungs after expiration. (From McKenry LM, Salerno E: *Mosby's Pharmacology in Nursing*, ed 18, St Louis, 1992, Mosby–Year Book.)

whereas some of the changes that occur with emphysema are irreversible. Chronic bronchitis and emphysema are often referred to as **chronic obstructive pulmonary disease (COPD)**. Asthma can be chronic, although it usually occurs more acutely and intermittently than COPD.[12] From time to time, various stressors, such as exposure to allergens or upper respiratory infections, can cause acute **exacerbations** of airway obstruction for COPD and asthma patients. These acute episodes are characterized by varying degrees of **bronchospasm**. Bronchospasm can lead to severe hypoxia requiring immediate attention. Figure 7-3 compares a bronchiole in a normal state with that of a bronchiole in spasm during an asthma attack.

Prehospital Management of Asthma

As with any patient demonstrating signs and symptoms of hypoxia, the initial intervention for the patient with asthma should be oxygen administration. Asthma-related deaths and serious complications, such as cardiac dysrhythmias and respiratory failure, are due primarily to hypoxia. The

MANAGEMENT OF ASTHMA IN PREGNANCY

Should the pregnant patient with an acute exacerbation of asthma be managed differently?

The administration of medication is always of great concern during pregnancy. The majority of the beta-adrenergic bronchodilators are FDA Category C. These drugs should be used when their potential benefits outweigh the risks of administration, as is the case in severe asthma. The hypoxemia that occurs in asthma is a significant threat to the well-being of both mother and fetus. Therefore, oxygen should be administered, and if necessary, a beta-agonist, such as albuterol, should be administered.

KEY TERMS

Bronchospasm—contraction of the smooth muscle of the bronchioles, resulting in acute narrowing of the airway lumen and obstruction to air flow; characterized by generalized wheezing.

Chronic obstructive pulmonary disease (COPD)—a progressive condition characterized by diminished ventilatory function; includes emphysema, bronchitis, and asthma.

method and concentration of oxygen administered depends on the severity of the illness. Administration of low-flow oxygen at 2 to 3 L/min via nasal cannula is appropriate for most asthmatic patients. Extreme cases may require that oxygen be administered via an endotracheal tube.

Bronchodilators

In addition to oxygen the major therapy for bronchospasm associated with asthma or COPD is the administration of a bronchodilating agent. Bronchodilators relax the smooth muscle of the tracheobronchial tree, resulting in increased opening of the bronchioles (bronchodilation) and decreased airway resistance. Classifications of bronchodilating agents pertinent to prehospital care presented in this chapter are sympathomimetic bronchodilating agents, xanthine derivatives, and anticholinergic agents.

Sympathomimetic bronchodilators. The sympathomimetic bronchodilating agents used in the prehospital setting are summarized in Table 7-2. These agents can be divided into two major groups. The first group includes epinephrine, a catecholamine that acts on alpha, beta$_1$- and beta$_2$-adrenergic receptors (see Chapter 6 for a detailed discussion of alpha and beta recep-

Table 7-2   Sympathomimetic Bronchodilators

DRUG NAME	PREPARATION	% USUAL ADULT DOSE	FDA PREGNANCY CATEGORY
Non-selective Sympathomimetic Bronchodilators			
Epinephrine (Adrenalin)	1:1000 solution for injection	0.1-0.5 mg subcutaneously	C
Beta$_2$-selective Sympathomimetic Bronchodilators			
Albuterol (Proventil, Ventolin)	Metered-dose inhaler Solution for nebulization (5 mg/ml)	2 inhalations (180 μg) q4h-6h 0.5 mg in 2-4 ml normal saline, administered over 5-15 minutes	C
Metaproterenol (Alupent, Metaprel)	Metered-dose inhaler Solution for nebulization (50 mg/ml)	2-3 inhalations (1.3-1.95 mg) 10-15 mg in 2-4 ml normal saline, administered over 5-15 minutes	C
Isoetharine (Bronkosol)	Metered-dose inhaler Solution for nebulization	1-2 inhalations (340 μg) Hand-nebulizer, 4-7 inhalations undiluted 1% solution	C
Terbutaline sulfate (Brethine)	Solution for injection	0.25 mg subcutaneously	B

FDA, Federal drug administration.

tors). Epinephrine is indicated in respiratory emergencies for its ability to stimulate beta$_2$-adrenergic receptors. Stimulation of beta$_2$-adrenergic receptors in the lungs causes dilation of airways by relaxing airway smooth muscle, decreasing chemical mediator release (such as histamine) and decreasing inflammation.

Although epinephrine has a long history of use in the treatment of acute bronchospasm, it has some disadvantages when compared with the more selective beta$_2$ agonists available today. Epinephrine's stimulation of alpha and beta$_1$ receptors causes undesirable effects, such as tremor, tachycardia, and dysrhythmias. Epinephrine administration increases myocardial oxygen demand by increasing heart rate, force of contraction, and peripheral vascular resistance. Most children and young adults tolerate this increase in myocardial oxygen demand well, but other patients, such as those with coronary artery disease, hypertension, or those over age 40, may develop myocardial ischemia when given epinephrine. Particularly for these patients, the more selective beta$_2$-adrenergic agonists discussed in the following paragraph are the appropriate drugs of choice for managing acute bronchospasm.

The second group of sympathomimetic bronchodilating agents are chemically related to epinephrine but are more selective for beta$_2$-adrenergic receptors. Current research and practice suggest that these are the preferred agents in the management of acute bronchospasm.[1,13,23] At therapeutic doses, these agents primarily stimulate beta$_2$-adrenergic receptors, resulting in bronchodilation without the undesired effects of beta$_1$ stimulation.

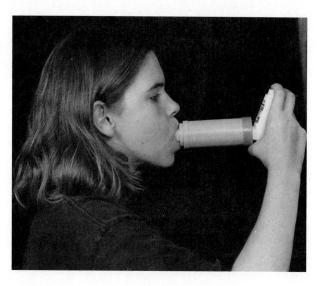

Figure 7-4   Metered-dose inhaler with a spacer device.

Patients receiving these agents are less likely to experience the muscle tremors and cardiac effects (e.g., tachycardia, ischemia, dysrhythmias) seen with epinephrine administration. Examples of these drugs include terbutaline sulfate, albuterol, metaproterenol, and isoetharine.

Albuterol, metaproterenol, and isoetharine are administered by **inhalation** in the form of aerosol therapy. An aerosol is a gas or solution in which fine liquid or solid particles are suspended. Aerosols are administered by **metered-dose inhalers** (Figure 7-4) or **nebulizers** (Figure 7-5). Today, aerosol administration of beta-agonists is the primary treatment for acute exacerbation of asthma and COPD in emergency settings.*

Aerosol administration offers several advantages over subcutaneous administration. Aerosol administration delivers the medication directly to the airway, which allows for smaller doses than would otherwise be required, and results in minimal systemic absorption and fewer side effects. Aerosol administration is also generally more comfortable for patients than subcutaneous injection, which is particularly important in children. A recent

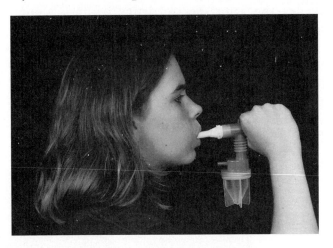

Figure 7-5   Hand-held nebulizer.

KEY TERMS

Metered-dose inhaler—a device for administering medications by inhalation; it consists of a canister containing a liquid, which, when activated, delivers the medication in a fine mist.

Nebulizer—a device that delivers liquid medication in a fine spray; nebulizers are usually powered by oxygen or compressed air.

---

*References 1, 2, 4, 8, 22, 23.

study demonstrates that albuterol can be safely and effectively administered in the prehospital setting using a hand-held nebulizer.[22] Patients in the study experienced statistically significant improvement in peak expiratory flow rates (which indicates decreased airway resistance) after albuterol administration.

Both metered-dose inhalers and nebulizers are currently being used in the field. The boxes below describe the administration of aerosols by metered-dose inhaler and hand-held nebulizer. Nebulizers deliver the medication over several minutes and are considered by many to be superior to metered-dose inhalers in acute, severe airflow obstruction.[17] As the bronchioles dilate, the medication is delivered deeper and deeper into the lungs. Another advantage is the ease of use and humidification provided by this method.

An advantage of the metered-dose inhaler is that it does not require an oxygen source and is administered quickly and easily. Equivalent bronchodilation can be achieved with metered-dose inhalers only if an adequate number of activations are administered. A recent study demonstrated that the jet

---

HOW TO CORRECTLY USE A METERED-DOSE INHALER

1. Shake the canister thoroughly.
2. Exhale through the nose.
3. Place mouth on mouthpiece, and inhale deeply while depressing the canister.*

4. Hold breath for a few seconds.
5. Exhale slowly.
6. Wait at least two minutes before repeating the dose.

*A *spacer* may be used with metered-dose inhalers. These devices are particularly useful in pediatric patients but can be used with other patients as well. The spacer acts as a reservoir for the medication when the canister is activated. The medication is then inhaled by the patient. Use of the spacer negates the need for precise timing of inhalation and activation of the canister and ensures that an accurate dose is delivered.

ADMINISTERING MEDICATION BY NEBULIZER

1. Place the medication in the medication reservoir.
2. Have the patient exhale.
3. Place the mouthpiece in the patient's mouth.

4. Have the patient inhale slowly and deeply.
5. Have the patient hold his breath for 1 to 2 seconds.
6. Repeat steps 2 through 5 until all the medication is used.

nebulizer and a metered-dose inhaler with a spacer device were equally effective in acute severe airflow obstruction.[17]

Subcutaneous administration of terbutaline or epinephrine provide an alternative to inhalation in patients who are unable to cooperate with aerosol administration, such as young children or patients with decreased levels of consciousness. Subcutaneous administration is also useful for patients in whom bronchospasm is so severe that they cannot move adequate amounts of air. For these patients the subcutaneous route can be used initially, and aerosol administration can be initiated once ventilation is increased.

Xanthine Derivatives. Xanthine derivatives are a group of drugs that includes caffeine, theophylline, and theobromine. Theophylline is the only xanthine derivative used in prehospital care. Aminophylline is an IV preparation of the drug theophylline, which, until recently, was considered an essential first-line agent in the treatment of acute asthma. Aminophylline was used extensively in the prehospital setting for its bronchodilating effects. Recent studies have shown, however, that aminophylline has little efficacy on the acute management of asthma, offers no apparent advantage over the beta-adrenergic agonists, and has potentially dangerous side effects.[7,9,10,19] Aminophylline has been shown to offer no additional benefit to beta$_2$-agonist therapy in the first 4 hours of treatment.[6,9] When given alone, it is 3 to 4 times less effective in relieving acute bronchospasm than the beta$_2$-agonists.[10] When given in combination with a beta$_2$-agonist, adverse effects are increased without improved bronchodilation.[9]

Another important consideration in using aminophylline is its potentially dangerous side effects, which include tachycardia, premature ventricular contractions, and increased myocardial oxygen consumption. It is recommended that aminophylline be withheld initially in hospitalized patients in favor of other, less toxic therapies, such as the beta$_2$-agonists.[20]

Although theophylline preparations still play an important role in the management of chronic asthma, the use of aminophylline in the emergency department and the prehospital setting has also been questioned. Some emergency services have, in fact, removed aminophylline from their inventories in favor of the less toxic, more selective beta$_2$-adrenergic agents.

Anticholinergic agents. Ipratropium bromide (Atrovent) is an anticholinergic agent administered by inhalation that is being used with increasing frequency in the emergency department. The bronchodilating effects of anticholinergic drugs have been recognized for many years, but their side effects significantly limited their use. However, when used in combination with a beta-adrenergic agonist, ipratropium, promotes bronchodilation with minimal side effects as a result of the low doses afforded by aerosol administration and the fact that ipratropium has little effect on the central nervous system.

Although ipratropium is not currently being used in the field, it is being used in the emergency department. Initial bronchodilation is seen in the first few minutes following administration, but peak effects are not seen for 1 to 2 hours, making ipratropium more appropriate for maintenance treatment than for acute exacerbation of asthma. Ipratropium should be administered in combination with or following the administration of a beta-adrenergic agonist.

Corticosteroids

Corticosteroids are valuable adjuncts in the treatment of severe asthma, although their exact mechanism of action is still an area of controversy. The administration of corticosteroids in asthma can improve the responsiveness of the airway muscles to beta-agonists, stabilize membranes of cells that produce chemical mediators (e.g., histamine), and act as direct antiinflammatory agents to reduce edema and prevent migration of inflammatory cells into the area. Corticosteroids do not dilate the airways directly.

There is some controversy related to the administration of corticosteroids in the field. The effects of corticosteroids can take several hours, so immediate improvement is not seen in the field. On the other hand it is important that they be administered early in the course of treatment. Patients most likely to benefit from corticosteroid administration are those currently taking steroids, those recently taken off steroids, those not responding to initial treatment with inhaled medications, and those with a history of severe disease.

Corticosteroids are given intravenously in the field. However, inhaled corticosteroids are effective for the treatment of asthma and are currently being used in the hospital setting and by patients at home. Corticosteroids are also indicated in the prehospital management of anaphylaxis. The corticosteroid most commonly used in prehospital care is methylprednisolone (Solu-Medrol).

Hydrocortisone sodium succinate (Hydrocortisone, Solu-Cortef) is a short-acting glucocorticosteroid with properties similar to those of methylprednisolone. Because it has more mineralocorticoid activity (e.g., fluid retention), it is used less frequently in the prehospital setting and emergency department than methylprednisolone.

ANAPHYLAXIS

Anaphylaxis is a sudden, severe response to the reexposure of an antigen (severe allergic reaction) and is mediated by specialized white blood cells (mast cells and basophils) that release chemical substances, the most important of which is histamine. The reaction may be local or systemic. The release of histamine causes dilation of capillaries, increased secretion of gastric juices, and contraction of smooth muscles of the bronchi and uterus.

Symptoms of severe systemic reactions can include laryngeal edema, bronchospasm, and circulatory collapse. The major goal of therapy in severe anaphylactic reactions is restoration of circulatory and respiratory function. Prehospital drug therapy for anaphylaxis most often includes the administration of oxygen and epinephrine. It may also include the administration of antihistamines and corticosteroids.

Epinephrine is the first-line drug in cases of anaphylaxis. It inhibits the release of histamine from the mast cells, restoring autonomic tone to the vessels and dilating the bronchioles.

Antihistamines antagonize the effects of histamine. Diphenhydramine hydrochloride (Benadryl) is the antihistamine used most frequently in the field. It may be ordered in addition to epinephrine.

Corticosteroids can also be used as an adjunct to epinephrine in anaphylactic reactions. Corticosteroids are valuable for their antiinflammatory effects.

SUMMARY

Respiratory emergencies require immediate recognition and action by paramedics. The major goal of treatment is to improve tissue oxygenation. Priority should be given to airway maintenance and oxygen administration. The method, flow rate, and concentration of oxygen are determined by the nature and severity of the patient's condition. The sympathomimetic bronchodilators play an important role in the treatment of respiratory emergencies. More specifically, beta$_2$-agonists administered by inhalation are currently the drugs of choice in respiratory emergencies associated with asthma and COPD.

In respiratory emergencies related to anaphylaxis, oxygen, epinephrine, antihistamines, and corticosteroids may be administered in the prehospital setting.

REFERENCES

1. Barnes PJ: Drug therapy—a new approach to the treatment of asthma, *Med Intell* 321(22):1517, 1989.
2. Brenner BE: Bronchial asthma in adults: presentation to the emergency department, part II: Sympathomimetics, respiratory failure, recommendations for initial treatment, indications for admission and summary, *Am J Emerg Med* 1:306, 1983.

3. Chameides L, editor: *Textbook of pediatric advanced life support*, American Heart Association, 24, 1988.

4. Eilers MA, Lander DH: COPD: update on a complex cardiorespiratory syndrome, *Emerg Med Rep* 7(20):153, 1986.

5. Fanta C, Rossing TH, McFadden ER: Glucocorticoids in acute asthma, a critical controlled trial, *Am J Med* 74:845, 1983.

6. *Guidelines for the diagnosis and management of asthma*, National asthma education program, August 1991, Publication No. 91-3042.

7. Josephson GW et al: Emergency treatment of asthma: a comparison of two regimens, *JAMA* 242(7):639, 1979.

8. Karkal SS, editor: Rapid amelioration of acute bronchospasm in pediatric asthma, *Emerg Med Rep* 10(23):185, 1989.

9. Kelly HW, Murphy S: Should we stop using theophylline for the treatment of the hospitalized patient with status asthmaticus? *DICP Ann Pharmacol* 32:995, 1989.

10. Littenberg B: Aminophylline treatment in severe acute asthma: a mega analysis, *JAMA* 259(11):1678, 1989.

11. Littenberg B, Gluck EH: A controlled trial of methylprednisolone in the emergency treatment of acute asthma, *N Engl J Med* 314(3):150, 1986.

12. McCance KL, Huether SE: *Pathophysiology: the biologic basis for disease in adults and children*, St Louis, 1990, Mosby–Year Book.

13. McFadden ER: Therapy of acute asthma, *J Allergy Clin Immunol* 84(2):151, 1989.

14. McKenry LM, Salerno E: *Pharmacology in nursing*, ed 18, St Louis, 1992, Mosby–Year Book.

15. Owens GR, Rogers RM: Managing respiratory failure in chronic airflow obstruction, *J Respir Dis* 3(7), July 1982.

16. Rossing TH et al: Emergency therapy of asthma: comparison of the acute effects of parenteral and inhaled sympathomimetics and infused aminophylline, *Am Rev Respir Dis* 122:365, 1980.

17. Salzman GA et al: Aerosolized metaproterenol in the treatment of asthmatics with severe airflow obstruction, comparison of two delivery methods, *Chest* 95(5):1017, 1989.

18. Schatz M et al: The safety of inhaled beta-agonist bronchodilators during pregnancy, *J Allerg Clin Immunol* 82(4):686, 1988.

19. Self TH et al: Is theophylline use justified in acute exacerbations of asthma? *Pharmacotherapy* 9(4):260, 1989.

20. Shrestha M et al: Decreased duration of emergency department treatment of chronic obstructive pulmonary disease exacerbations with the addition of ipratropium bromide to beta-agonist therapy, *Ann Emerg Med* 20(11):1206, 1991.

21. Summer W et al: Aerosol bronchodilator delivery methods, *Arch Intern Med* 149:618, 1989.

22. Vonderohe EA et al: The prehospital use of albuterol inhalation treatment, *Prehosp Disast Med* 6(3):327, 1991.

23. Young G, Gliden D: Acute bronchospasm, *Emerg Med Serv* 32(1):28, 1992.

DRUG PROFILES
◆ Albuterol Sulfate (Proventil, Ventolin)

Albuterol is a direct-acting sympathomimetic bronchodilator. Its bronchodilating actions are similar to those of epinephrine, but like terbutaline sulfate, it has greater selectivity for beta$_2$-adrenergic receptors than beta$_1$-adrenergic receptors.

Mechanism of action

Albuterol acts directly on the beta$_2$-adrenergic receptors to relax bronchial smooth muscle, resulting in reduced airway resistance and relief of bronchospasm.

Indications

Albuterol is indicated in the relief of bronchospasm in patients with reversible obstructive airway disease, such as bronchial asthma and in acute exacerbation of COPD.

Contraindication

- hypertension

Precautions

Although albuterol reportedly produces less cardiac stimulation than other sympathomimetics, it should nonetheless be used with great caution in any patient with known cardiovascular disease. Safety in pregnancy is established at FDA Category C.

Side effects

- headache
- drowsiness
- dizziness
- nausea

Interactions

Monoamine oxidase inhibitors and tricyclic antidepressants may increase the potential for cardiovascular adverse reactions. Although it is acceptable to administer albuterol while the patient is on other sympathomimetic agents, the patient should be observed for additive interaction. Propranolol and other beta-blockers may antagonize the effects of albuterol.

Dosage

Adults: Inhaler—1 to 2 inhalations (90 µg each), may be repeated every 15 minutes as needed. Nebulizer—0.5 ml (2.5 mg) in 2 to 4 ml of normal saline over 5 to 15 minutes.

Children: Nebulizer—0.03 ml/kg of a 5% solution up to 1.0 ml over 5 to 10 minutes.

Administration

Albuterol is supplied in a solution for nebulization and in a metered-dose inhaler.

◆ Aminophylline

Aminophylline has been used for many years in respiratory emergencies for its bronchodilating properties. Several recent studies have shown no benefit and possibly increased adverse effects in the management of acute bronchospasm. Many practitioners no longer recommend its use routinely.

Mechanism of action

Aminophylline directly relaxes the smooth muscle of the bronchi, resulting in the reversal of bronchospasm caused by acute and chronic asthma, bronchitis, and emphysema. Other pulmonary effects include stimulation of the respiratory center, reduction in pulmonary hypertension and alveolar carbon dioxide tension, and increased pulmonary blood flow. Aminophylline also reduces diaphragmatic muscle fatigue, stimulates the central nervous system, promotes diuresis, increases secretion of gastric acid, and increases heart rate and force of contraction.

Indications

Aminophylline can be useful in bronchospasm associated with asthma, chronic bronchitis, or emphysema and bronchospasm associated with congestive heart failure or pulmonary edema.

Contraindications

Allergy or hypersensitivity to xanthine compounds.

Precautions

Caution should be used when administering aminophylline to patients with angina, preexisting dysrhythmias, peptic ulcer disease, liver disease, or renal disease. Aminophylline should not be administered to children under 6 months of age. Aminophylline has a narrow margin of safety with a high potential for toxicity, especially if given too rapidly by IV. Because side effects are dose-dependent, flow rates should be carefully monitored. The patient's heart rate and rhythm should be monitored throughout the administration of aminophylline. Aminophylline should not be given as prehospital therapy to patients who are on oral preparations of theophylline. Aminophylline is usually not administered in the emergency department until serum levels are determined. Safety in pregnancy is established at FDA Category C.

Side effects

Side effects increase in frequency when serum levels rise above therapeutic levels. Side effects include flushing, nausea, vomiting, diarrhea, irritability, tremors, headache, and insomnia. As serum levels continue to rise, tachycardia, other cardiac dysrhythmias, hypotension, seizures, brain damage, and death can occur.

Interactions

Many drugs can interact with aminophylline. Aminophylline increases the patient's sensitivity to digitalis toxicity. Furosemide and propranolol increase the effects of aminophylline. Smoking decreases the effects of aminophylline.

Dosage

Adults: 6 mg/kg not to exceed 20 mg/min, usually over 20 to 30 minutes as a loading dose, followed by a maintenance dose of 0.5 to 0.9 mg/kg per hour by infusion.

Children: 6 to 8 mg/kg not to exceed 20 mg/min, usually over 20 to 30 minutes as a loading dose, followed by a maintenance dose of 1 mg/kg per hour by infusion.

Administration

In respiratory emergencies aminophylline is administered by IV infusion, mixed in 50 to 250 ml of D$_5$W. The infusion rate should never exceed a rate of 20 mg/min. Rapid infusion can result in hypotension and circulatory collapse. Aminophylline is available for IV use in 250- and 500-mg ampules.

◆ Diphenhydramine Hydrochloride (Benadryl)

Diphenhydramine is the most commonly used antihistamine in the prehospital setting. It is used for respiratory distress associated with anaphylaxis.

Mechanism of action

Diphenhydramine blocks the effect of histamine in allergic reactions, inhibits motion sickness, and causes sedation.

Indications

Diphenhydramine is used as an adjunct therapy to epinephrine in anaphylaxis and severe allergic reaction. It is also used for mild to moderate allergic reactions.

Contraindications

- Asthma is a relative contraindication depending on its severity. Diphenhydramine should not be administered in severe, uncontrolled asthma.
- narrow-angle glaucoma
- prostatic hypertrophy

Precautions

Safety for use in pregnancy has not been established.

Side effects

- drowsiness, dizziness, incoordination, confusion
- dry mouth
- drying of bronchial secretions
- blurred vision
- urinary retention

Interactions

Diphenhydramine may cause additive central nervous system depression when given with other central nervous system depressants.

Dosage

Diphenhydramine is available in ampules and prefilled syringes containing 50 mg in 1 ml.
Adults: The usual dosage is 10 to 50 mg intravenously or intramuscularly.
Children: 1 to 2 mg/kg intravenously or intramuscularly.

Administration

Diphenhydramine is administered intramuscularly or intravenously in the emergency setting. Oral preparations are available for less emergent use.

◆ Epinephrine (Adrenalin) See page 189.

◆ Ipratropium Bromide (Atrovent)

Ipratropium bromide is an anticholinergic drug.

Mechanism of action

Ipratropium bromide causes bronchodilation by competitive inhibition of cholinergic receptors on bronchial smooth muscle.

Indications

- used in combination with other bronchodilators in the treatment of chronic asthma
- may be used in acute exacerbations of asthma in combination with beta-adrenergic agonists

Contraindications

None.

Precautions

Ipratropium can cause bronchoconstriction to worsen. This is thought to be related to the hypotonicity of the solution or to additives, such as benzalkonium chloride.[1] It is for this reason that beta-adrenergic agonists should be given first or in combination with ipratropium.

Side effects

Side effects are uncommon because there is little systemic absorption of ipratropium bromide. Patients may experience a transient dryness of mouth, scratchy throat, or bitter taste.

Interactions

Ipratropium has been used with other drugs including sympathomimetic bronchodilators, methylxanthines, and corticosteroids without adverse reactions.

Dosage

The usual dose is 36 μg (two inhalations).

Administration

Ipratropium is administered by inhalation. It is available for use in metered-dose inhalers or given by nebulizer.

◆ Methylprednisolone (Solu-Medrol)

Methylprednisolone is an intermediate-acting, synthetic corticosteroid with potent antiinflammatory properties.

Mechanism of action

Methylprednisolone suppresses acute and chronic inflammation and potentiates the beta-adrenergic's relaxation of smooth muscle.

Indications

- acute exacerbation of reactive airway disease (asthma and COPD)
- respiratory distress associated with anaphylaxis
- other allergic reactions
- spinal injury

Contraindications

There are no contraindications to a single dose.

Precautions

None in emergency administration of a single dose.

Side effects

The side effects of corticosteroids are vast and occur most often with long-term use. The most notable are sodium and water retention, gastrointestinal problems, and steroid-induced diabetes mellitus. There are no significant side effects associated with a single dose used in emergencies.

Interactions

Can potentiate hypokalemia when given with diuretics.

Dosage

Adults: The dosage range of methylprednisolone is 10 to 250 mg, with the common adult dose being 80 to 125 mg. May be repeated every 4 to 8 hours.

Children: 30 mg/kg can be used in high-dose therapy. The dose can be reduced in infants and children but should not be less than 0.5 mg/kg in 24 hours.

Administration

In emergency settings methylprednisolone is administered intravenously. Rapid administration of large doses can result in hypotension and cardiovascular collapse. Administration should be slow (250 mg/0.5 min).

◆ Oxygen

Oxygen is an odorless, colorless, and tasteless gas normally present in the atmosphere at a concentration of about 21%.

Mechanism of action

The administration of oxygen increases the concentration of oxygen delivered to the alveoli, which in turn increases the amount of oxygen in the blood available for transport to the tissues.

Indications

Oxygen is indicated in any situation in which tissue hypoxia is likely to occur, including but not limited to:
- ischemic chest pain
- dyspnea
- shock
- significant hemorrhage
- congestive heart failure
- multiple trauma
- inhalation of toxic substances, such as carbon monoxide or chlorine gas
- near drowning
- burns
- head injury

Contraindications

There are no contraindications in emergent situations. (One exception to this is the ingestion of the herbicides paraquat or diaquat. Oxygen potentiates the toxicity of these agents. Poisoning from these substances in the United States is uncommon.)

Precautions

Oxygen should be used cautiously in patients who are known to have COPD.

Side effects

In emergent situations oxygen can generally be administered without harmful effects.

Interactions

None.

Dosage

The dosage of oxygen is determined by the patient's underlying condition. Generally, in emergent situations oxygen should be given at the highest concentration available.

Administration

Oxygen is administered by inhalation. The specific method of delivery depends on the patient's underlying problem (see chapter text).

◆ Terbutaline Sulfate (Brethine)

Terbutaline is a synthetic sympathomimetic bronchodilator. Its actions are similar to those of epinephrine, but it has greater selectivity for beta$_2$-adrenergic receptors.

Mechanism of action

Terbutaline relaxes smooth muscle of the tracheobronchial tree by stimulating beta$_2$-adrenergic receptors. It provides bronchodilation with minimal cardiac effect (i.e., alpha and beta$_1$ effects).

Indications

- bronchial asthma
- bronchospasm associated with emphysema and bronchitis

Contraindications

- hypersensitivity
- tachycardia (tachycardia is considered a relative contraindication because it may be related to hypoxia and may resolve with improved ventilation)

Precautions

Administration of terbutaline can lower the diastolic blood pressure. Cardiovascular effects are more frequent with subcutaneous administration than with oral administration. Safety has not been demonstrated for children under 12 years of age. As with all sympathomimetics, the patient's cardiac rhythm and vital signs should be monitored carefully. Safety in pregnancy is established at FDA Category B.

Side effects

The side effects of terbutaline are usually mild and are dose-related. They are similar to the side effects seen with other sympathomimetics. Side effects include restlessness, apprehension, tremor, dizziness, palpitations, tachycardia, dysrhythmias, and increased or decreased blood pressure.

Interactions

Terbutaline can increase the cardiovascular effects of other sympathomimetic drugs. Beta-blockers antagonize the effect of terbutaline.

Dosage

Adults: Subcutaneously—0.25 mg; may be repeated in 15 to 30 minutes, not to exceed 0.5 mg in 4 hours. Inhalation—400 µg.

Children: Although manufacturers indicate that safety has not been established in children under 12 years of age, terbutaline is given to children in practice. Medical direction and local protocols should be consulted for dosage.

Administration

Terbutaline is most often administered subcutaneously in the prehospital setting. The onset of action when given subcutaneously is 5 to 15 minutes. Peak action occurs in 30 minutes. Terbutaline is available in a 1 mg/ml solution. Terbutaline can also be administered by inhalation.

8

Cardiovascular Emergencies

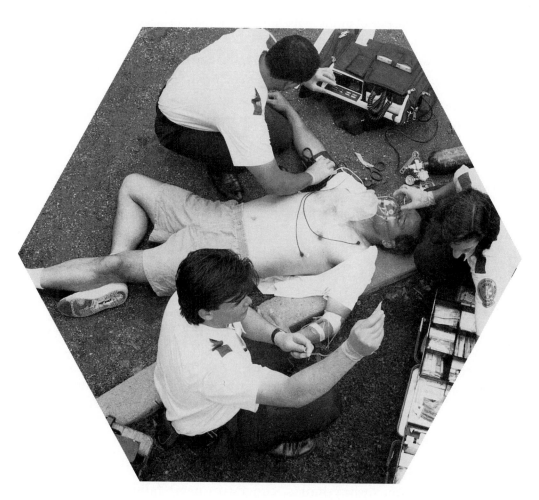

OBJECTIVES

1. Describe the significance of cardiovascular emergencies in prehospital care.
2. Describe the prehospital management of chest pain.
3. Name the drug of choice for the treatment of pain associated with angina pectoris.
4. Describe the benefits of using morphine sulfate for pain associated with myocardial infarction.
5. Explain the role of thrombolytic agents in the prehospital setting.
6. List the cardiac dysrhythmias for which drugs are commonly administered in the prehospital setting.
7. Differentiate among the different types of antidysrhythmic drugs.
8. List the actions, indications, and major side effects of the commonly used antidysrhythmic drugs.
9. Explain the role of medications in the prehospital management of congestive heart failure and pulmonary edema.
10. Describe the use of catecholamines in cardiac arrest.
11. Explain the use of atropine in symptomatic bradycardias.
12. Describe the prehospital management of hypertensive emergencies.
13. Explain the role of the American Heart Association in Advanced Cardiac Life Support.

Cardiovascular emergencies are frequently encountered by paramedics and require a variety of interventions, including advanced airway management, IV, and electrical therapy. The administration of medications also plays an integral role in the prehospital management of cardiovascular emergencies.

Drugs used for cardiovascular emergencies are given primarily for their effects on one or more of the following: heart rate, heart rhythm, contractility, myocardial oxygen demand, and peripheral vascular resistance. The American Heart Association (AHA) has developed guidelines for administering these drugs for advanced cardiac life support (ACLS) and pediatric advanced life support (PALS). These guidelines reflect a consensus of an interdisciplinary group of experts. As such, these are considered the most effective guidelines that current knowledge and experience can provide.[6,7] The information presented in this chapter is consistent with AHA guidelines.

This chapter covers drug therapy for patients with chest pain, myocardial infarction, dysrhythmias, congestive heart failure, and hypertension.

DRUGS PROFILED IN THIS CHAPTER

CLASSIFICATION	DRUG	PAGE
Alkalinizing agent	Sodium bicarbonate	199
Anticholinergic	Atropine sulfate	183
Antidysrhythmic	Adenosine	180
	Bretylium tosylate	184
	Lidocaine hydrochloride	193
	Procainamide hydrochloride	197
Calcium Channel Blockers	Nifedipine	195
	Verapamil	200
Diuretic	Furosemide	191
Nitrate	Nitroglycerin	196
Sympathomimetic	Dobutamine hydrochloride	186
	Dopamine	187
	Epinephrine	189
	Isoproterenol	192
Thrombolytic	Recombinant alteplase	181

The major drug groups discussed are nitrates, thrombolytics, antidysrhythmics, sympathomimetics, anticholinergics, cardiac glycosides, diuretics, and calcium channel blockers. To understand the information presented in this chapter, students should be familiar with key terms related to cardiac function (see box on page 164).

◆ CASE PRESENTATIONS

Case Presentation 1 (Myocardial Infarction)

At 10:30 AM one Monday, MEDIC 8 is called to a local corporate office for a "possible heart attack." They arrive in 12 minutes to find a 47-year-old male complaining of severe, left-sided substernal chest pain radiating down his left arm. One of the paramedics places the patient on oxygen via a nasal cannula at 6 L/min. Her partner places the ECG electrodes on the patient's chest. The patient's vital signs are: P-84 and irregular,

KEY TERMS RELATED TO CARDIAC FUNCTION

Absolute refractory—referring to that interval of time following depolarization during which the cell is incapable of responding to another stimulus.

Afterload—the pressure against which the ventricle has to contract to eject its contents; increased arterial pressure increases afterload.

Automaticity—the property of the cells of the heart's conducting system whereby an impulse is initiated without outside stimulation; self-excitation or self-depolarization.

Cardiac output (CO)—the volume of blood pumped by the heart per minute (about 5 liters in average adult); cardiac output is a function of stroke volume (SV) and heart rate (HR) and is represented by the formula SV × HR = CO.

Chronotropic—referring to a drug's effect on heart rate; when a drug is said to have a positive chronotropic effect, it results in an increase in heart rate; a negative chronotropic effect refers to a decrease in heart rate.

Conduction—the transmission of impulses from one cardiac cell to another.

Conduction velocity—the speed with which impulses are transmitted from one cell to another.

Depolarization—the process by which cardiac contraction is initiated; it is accomplished by the movement of electrolytes across the cell membrane and a change in the electrical charge of the cell membrane.

Dromotropic—referring to a drug's effect on conduction velocity; a positive dromotropic effect refers to an increase in conduction velocity: a negative dromotropic effect refers to a decrease in conduction velocity.

Excitability—the ability of a cell to respond to an electrical stimulus.

Inotropic—referring to a drug's effect on the heart's force of contraction; when a drug is said to have a positive inotropic effect, it results in an increased force of contraction; a negative chronotropic effect refers to a decrease in the force of contraction.

Preload—the amount (volume) of blood in the ventricle at the end of diastole; as venous return increases, preload increases; increased preload is accompanied by increased stretch on the myocardial muscle, resulting in increased force of contraction in the normal heart.

Relative refractory—relative refractory is that period of time during which a stronger stimulus than normal is required to elicit a response.

Repolarization—return of the cell to its resting state.

Stroke volume (SV)—the amount of blood ejected by the ventricle with each contraction.

R-16, and BP-140/90. The cardiac monitor indicates that he is in normal sinus rhythm with frequent, multifocal premature ventricular contractions and several runs of ventricular tachycardia.

The paramedic asks, "How long have you had this pain?" She notes he is slightly diaphoretic and grimaces as he reponds. He indicates his chest pain began about 30 minutes earlier and became progressively worse. She auscultates his chest and hears clear breath sounds.

The history indicates that the patient has angina but perceives this episode of pain to be more severe. The patient reports having no allergies and having taken two nitroglycerin tablets before the paramedics arrived.

After explaining that she is going to give him another nitroglycerin tablet, the paramedic places it under his tongue. She explains that they also want to start an IV. An IV of D_5W is initiated at a keep-open rate, and a 1 mg/kg bolus of lidocaine HCl is administered IV. The paramedics plan to follow with a second bolus of 0.5 mg/kg of lidocaine in 5 minutes. They prepare a lidocaine infusion by injecting 1 g of lidocaine into 250 ml D_5W, labeling the IV bag, and "piggybacking" the administration set into the primary IV line.

One of the paramedics contacts medical direction and gives the patient report. She receives orders to administer up to 4 mg of morphine sulfate in 2-mg increments and obtain a 12-lead ECG. If the ECG indicates an acute myocardial infarction, they are to send the ECG via ultrahigh frequency telemeter and prepare to administer alteplase. They are also to administer nitrous oxide if the patient's pain persists. The 4 mg of morphine sulfate is given, and the second bolus of lidocaine is administered.

The 12-lead ECG indicates that the patient is experiencing an acute anterior wall myocardial infarction, and the machine's automatic interpretation validates the paramedic's interpretation. She prepares to administer alteplase en route to the hospital.

Case Presentation 2 (Cardiac Arrest)

You are covering a local college football game when you hear cries for help in the stands. People in the crowd are waving at you, and you see someone starting CPR. A woman shouts to you, "He's my husband. He had two heart attacks in the past year." The patient appears to weigh approximately 100 kg and looks about 50 years old.

You follow the standing orders for cardiac arrest. A "quick look" reveals ventricular fibrillation. You charge the defibrillator to 200 joules and defibrillate. Your partner is preparing to administer positive-pressure ventilation and oxygen.

The patient's rhythm doesn't change with the first shock, so you defibrillate again, this time at 300 joules. His rhythm doesn't change, and you defibrillate at 360 joules.

You intubate the patient and prepare to administer 2 mg of a 1:1000 aqueous solution of epinephrine down the endotracheal tube. You request that your partner initiate an IV and then resume CPR and ventilations. There is no change in rhythm after the administration of epinephrine, so you defibrillate at 360 joules again. The patient remains in ventricular fibrillation. Lidocaine, 150 mg (1.5 mg/kg), is administered IV. You defibrillate at 360 joules once again, after which the ECG indicates a junctional bradycardia of 42 per minute.

The patient has a faint radial pulse and spontaneous shallow respirations of 12 per minute. His blood pressure is 84/62. You administer 1 mg of atropine IV, and the rhythm doesn't change. You contact medical direction to report on your progress and request additional orders for external pacing. Medical direction orders an external pacemaker at a rate of 70 beats per minute. The pacer captures, and the patient's level of consciousness and blood pressure improve.

Your crew prepares the patient for transport by moving him onto the stretcher and CPR board. The patient is transported to the nearest medical facility.

Case Presentation 3 (Congestive Heart Failure)

At 3:16 AM, MEDIC 6 receives a call from a patient with difficulty breathing. The paramedics arrive to find an elderly female whom they have transported on several occasions.

The patient turns her head slightly toward you—mostly just her eyes—as you enter the bedroom. She denies having chest pain, but you can hear the gurgling sound of fluid in her lungs as she struggles with each breath. You observe central cyanosis and profuse diaphoresis. Her vital signs are: P-92 (weak, thready), R-32, and BP-94/50.

You place her on high-flow oxygen by nonrebreather face mask and initiate an IV of D₅W at a keep-open rate. Medical direction orders 40 mg of furosemide IV and morphine sulfate 2 mg IV. You administer the medications and transport the patient to the nearest hospital. Reassessment while en route shows that the patient's dyspnea has lessened and breath sounds have improved. ◆

DRUGS USED IN THE MANAGEMENT OF CHEST PAIN

Nitrates

Chest pain of cardiac origin is caused by myocardial ischemia and is usually associated with angina pectoris, myocardial infarction, or dysrhythmias.

Angina pectoris is a condition characterized by chest pain and associated with inadequate oxygenation of the myocardium. Most angina is related to **atherosclerosis**. Atherosclerotic plaque causes the lumen of the coronary arteries to narrow, decreasing blood flow to myocardial tissue. When the oxygen demand of the myocardium exceeds the oxygen supply (typically with exercise, emotional stress, or extreme cold), chest pain occurs. Vasomotor spasm (vasospasm) is another less frequent cause of angina pectoris.

Anginal pain is usually described as a sudden, crushing, substernal pain. The pain may radiate to the left shoulder and down the left arm or into the jaw or neck area, and is frequently associated with a feeling of suffocation, nausea, and shortness of breath.

The drug of choice in the emergency management of anginal pain is nitroglycerin, which has been the cornerstone of therapy for anginal pain for more than 100 years.[10] Nitroglycerin belongs to a group of drugs called *nitrates* and is also referred to as an antianginal agent. Nitrates exert their effect on anginal pain by causing vasodilation.

A common misconception is that nitrates work primarily by dilating the coronary arteries, thereby improving blood flow to the myocardium. However, when coronary arteries are narrowed by atherosclerosis and calcification, they cannot adequately respond to vasodilators. Instead, these vasodilators exert their major therapeutic effect by causing peripheral vasodilation. Peripheral vasodilation causes a decrease in venous return to the heart and lowers the vascular resistance against which the heart must pump. Ultimately, the workload of the heart is reduced, and oxygen requirements are decreased.

Many dose forms of nitroglycerin exist, including oral preparations, transdermal patches, and topical ointments. Some of these forms have a long-term, sustained release and have little effect when immediate relief is needed. The dosage forms that provide for immediate relief of anginal pain are sublingual tablets, lingual aerosol metered-dose sprays, and liquid for IV use. IV administration of nitroglycerin is rarely used in the prehospital management of chest pain but may be encountered during the interhospital transport of patients with persistent chest pain that does not respond to other medications. Sublingual tablets are in common use today. Recently, a lingual aerosol form of nitroglycerin has been used safely and effectively in the prehospital setting.[23]

When administered sublingually, the onset of action of nitroglycerin is rapid. It is generally accepted that a total of three doses of nitroglycerin at 5-minute intervals may be administered, after which other interventions should be considered. The patient in Case Presentation 1 was given 3 doses of nitroglycerin without improvement. The paramedics acted appropriately in requesting orders for morphine.

It is often difficult to differentiate anginal pain from pain caused by myocardial infarction (MI). In MI, myocardial tissue becomes necrotic from severe, prolonged ischemia. If chest pain is not relieved with nitroglycerin, MI should be suspected. The relief of chest pain is especially important because chest pain causes an increase in circulating catecholamines, resulting in increased heart rate and force of contraction and, thus, myocardial oxygen consumption.

Analgesics

Morphine sulfate is the drug of choice for chest pain associated with MI. In addition to being a potent analgesic, morphine causes peripheral vasodilation, which reduces myocardial workload. Nitrous oxide can also be used in the treatment of chest pain. See drug profiles for morphine and nitrous oxide on pages 260 and 261, respectively.

THROMBOLYSIS

Thrombus (clot) formation frequently occurs in coronary arteries within the first few hours following the onset of symptoms of acute MI. The lysis, or dissolution, of occlusion-causing thrombi in coronary arteries is important in the treatment of acute MI. The fact that early administration of thrombolytic agents can prevent myocardial muscle damage has generated great interest in the administration of these agents in the prehospital setting.[13,27] There are two thrombolytic agents in current use: recombinant alteplase (Activase), commonly referred to as tissue plasminogen activator (tPA), and streptokinase. In the United States, tPA has been the thrombolytic agent of choice, whereas streptokinase is most often used in Europe.[9]

Timely administration of thrombolytic agents can reduce infarct size, improve ventricular function, and decrease mortality rates. Tissue plasminogen activator is currently being administered in clinical trials by several emergency medical services (EMS) organizations. It is of particular importance when transport times are long. Muscle damage occurs over time; prompt restoration of circulation reduces muscle damage. Because many patients may have experienced chest pain for several hours before seeking assistance from EMS, time can be critical. Local protocols for the administration of tPA vary, but a critical component is the necessity to transmit a 12-lead ECG to medical direction for determination of ECG changes consistent with MI. Thrombolytic therapy holds great promise, but continued research is needed to better define its implications for prehospital medicine.

DRUGS USED TO CONTROL HEART RATE AND RHYTHM

Any abnormality in the rate or rhythm of the heart is referred to as a dysrhythmia. The term arrhythmia is synonymous with dysrhythmia, and the two are often used interchangeably. For the purposes of this text the term dysrhythmia is used.

Dysrhythmias are the result of: (1) disturbances in automaticity, (2) disturbances in conductivity, or (3) a combination of both.[26] Dysrhythmias are usually classified by their site of origin and their rate. The clinical significance of the various dysrhythmias range from benign, or requiring no intervention, to life-threatening dysrhythmias that require prompt recognition and management.

The most common and certainly the most serious dysrhythmias that occur after acute MI are ventricular: premature ventricular contractions (PVCs), ventricular tachycardia (VT), and ventricular fibrillation (VF). Recognition of these dysrhythmias and appropriate intervention by prehospital personnel can significantly influence survival for victims of acute MI.

The dysrhythmias for which drugs are most often administered in the field include symptomatic bradycardias, supraventricular tachycardia (SVT), PVCs,VT, VF, third-degree (complete) heart block, asystole, and pulseless electrical activity (PEA) (see box on page 170). Although most dysrhythmias are seen in patients with cardiac disease, they can also result from hypoxia, electrocution, trauma, endocrine emergencies, drug toxicity, electrolyte disturbances, and numerous other conditions.

The AHA has developed algorithms, which provide a guide for prioritizing the various interventions required to manage specific dysrhythmias or cardiac arrest (see Appendix A). These interventions include CPR, endotracheal intubation, IV therapy, electrical therapy, and drug therapy. Among the drugs recommended for the various dysrhythmias are antidysrhythmics, catecholamines, and anticholinergics.

DYSRHYTHMIAS THAT REQUIRE PHARMACOLOGIC INTERVENTION IN THE PREHOSPITAL SETTING

- **Sinus bradycardia**—by definition a heart rate of less than 60. Sinus bradycardias are treated only when the patient becomes symptomatic (e.g., hypotension, loss of consciousness, or chest pain).

- **Supraventricular tachycardia (SVT)**—a dysrhythmia originating above the ventricle and characterized by a very rapid rate (>150).

- **Premature ventricular contraction (PVC)**—a contraction originating below the atrioventricular (AV) junction, occurring earlier than the next expected contraction, and characterized by a wider bizarre QRS complex. PVCs are significant because they represent an irritable (ischemic) focus in the ventricle.

- **Ventricular tachycardia (VT)**—a dysrhythmia originating in the ventricle, usually from a single focus characterized by a rapid ventricular rate and a wide, bizarre QRS. VT is a life-threatening dysrhythmia.

- **Ventricular fibrillation (VF)**—a lethal dysrhythmia in which numerous individual cardiac cells within the ventricle initiate electrical impulses, resulting in a chaotic twitching or quivering of the ventricle. (There is no cardiac output in VF.)

- **Atrioventricular (AV) block**—partial or complete interruption in the conduction of impulses in the AV node. (The clinical significance of an AV block is its effect on heart rate. Symptomatic bradycardias may occur with second- and third-degree AV block.)

- **Asystole**—a complete lack of electrical activity in the heart.

- **Pulseless electrical activity (PEA)**—a term used to describe dysrhythmias associated with organized electrical activity without a palpable pulse.[6]

CARDIAC ARREST IN INFANTS AND CHILDREN

Cardiac arrest in infants and children usually occurs as the result of progressive deterioration in respiratory and circulatory function. Primary cardiac events are rare. The drugs used in pediatric cardiovascular emergencies are essentially the same drugs used for adults. The preferred routes of drug administration for infants and children in cardiac arrest are IV and intraosseous. The endotracheal route can be used for those medications approved for endotracheal administration in the absence of IV or intraosseous access. Appendix B provides a decision tree for the management of bradycardia and asystole/pulseless arrest in pediatric patients, and a dosage chart for drugs used in pediatric cardiopulmonary resuscitation and post-resuscitation stabilization.

Case Presentation 2 illustrates the appropriate sequencing of interventions for patients in cardiac arrest. The patient's condition required the administration of a catecholamine (epinephrine) and an antidysrhythmic (lidocaine) for ventricular fibrillation. An anticholinergic (atropine) was administered to increase heart rate after a spontaneous rhythm was returned.

Sodium bicarbonate, an alkalinizing agent, has historically been used to combat the hypoxic acidosis that occurs in prolonged cardiopulmonary arrest. It is no longer used routinely in cardiac arrest and may, in fact, worsen outcome. It may be considered if the arrest period is prolonged and the patient is not intubated.

Antidysrhythmics

One of the most dramatic benefits of prehospital medicine has been the increased survival rate for patients with MIs and other critical cardiac events. The cornerstone of this evolution has been the ability of first-response emergency personnel to recognize and definitively treat lethal dysrhythmias, which are the most frequent cause of death following an MI.[6] Table 8-1 lists antidysrhythmics commonly used in the field and the dysrhythmias for which they are indicated.

Lidocaine is the most commonly used antidysrhythmic in the prehospital setting. Lidocaine decreases electrical conduction in ischemic or injured

Table 8-1 Antidysrhythmic Drugs Commonly Used in the Field and the Dysrhythmias for Which They are Indicated

DRUG	INDICATION
Adenosine	Paroxysmal supraventricular atrial tachycardia (PSVT)
Lidocaine	Premature ventricular contractions Ventricular tachycardia Ventricular fibrillation
Bretylium	Ventricular tachycardia Ventricular fibrillation
Atropine	Symptomatic bradycardias Asystole that does not respond to epinephrine
Epinephrine	Asystole Ventricular tachycardia (pulseless) Ventricular fibrillation Pulseless electrical activity

cardiac tissue without adversely affecting normal conduction.[23] Lidocaine raises the fibrillation threshold and decreases automaticity, thereby suppressing ventricular dysrhythmias. Lidocaine has little effect on conduction velocity and does not depress myocardial contractility. Consequently, there is usually no adverse effect on cardiac output or blood pressure.

Lidocaine is the drug of choice in the treatment of ventricular dysrhythmias, including VT, VF, and malignant PVCs (see box below). Lidocaine, however, is not indicated in torsades de pointes, an atypical form of VT. (The bottom box below describes the management of this condition.)

TREATING PREMATURE VENTRICULAR CONTRACTION

Isolated, infrequent PVCs require no treatment. Treatment is initiated when PVCs occur as follows (such PVCs are often referred to as malignant PVCs):
- more than six unifocal PVCs per minute
- multifocal PVCs
- couplets (two PVCs together)
- three or more PVCs in a row (defined as VT)
- R-on-T phenomenom (ectopic beats occurring very close to the T-wave of the previous QRS complex)

TORSADES DE POINTES

Torsades de pointes (TDP) is a relatively rare, atypical, irregular form of VT. Literally, torsades de pointes means "the twisting of the points" and is characterized by complexes that appear negative and then positive on the ECG. It is associated with a prolonged QT interval (LQT). LQT may be acquired and is generally associated with electrolyte imbalances or drugs. LQT may also be congenital. Although TDP tends to be rapid and terminate spontaneously, it may deteriorate into VF.

Lidocaine, which is usually administered in VT, can actually worsen TDP. For those patients with acquired LQT, IV administration of magnesium sulfate has been shown to be effective in the management of TDP for patients who are stable enough not to require electrical cardioversion. For those patients who require cardioversion and convert to a normal sinus rhythm, increasing the heart rate by administering atropine or isuprel can prevent its recurrence. For those patients with congenital LQT, management depends on beta-blockers. In prehospital management, distinguishing acquired LQT from congenital LQT is difficult, so magnesium sulfate is recommended.[18]

Because lidocaine exerts little effect on the AV node and atrial myocardium, it is of little or no use in the treatment of supraventricular dysrhythmias.

Lidocaine has been shown to reduce the incidence of VF in patients with acute MI and has been administered prophylactically in many EMS organizations. However, the toxic-to-therapeutic balance of lidocaine is delicate, and prophylactic use in uncomplicated MI is controversial.[6,25,26] The AHA no longer recommends prophylactic administration of lidocaine in uncomplicated acute MI or ischemia without PVCs.

Great care should be taken when administering lidocaine in patients with heart rates lower than 60. The bradycardia should be treated first, as the ventricular ectopy can be an escape rhythm resulting from a low heart rate. In this situation it would be very dangerous to eradicate the escape rhythm as this will further decrease cardiac output.

Lidocaine is usually initially administered by IV bolus, followed by IV infusion. Specific dosing regimens are covered in the drug profile at the end of this chapter. It is important to recognize that lidocaine is also used as a topical anesthetic agent; however, only lidocaine that has been specially prepared for cardiac use can be administered intravenously. Only lidocaine that has been prepared without preservatives or epinephrine should be used, and the label should read "IV use for cardiac dysrhythmias."

Procainamide hydrochloride (Pronestyl), an antidysrhythmic similar to lidocaine, decreases cardiac excitability and automaticity and slows conduction velocity. It is indicated in recurrent VT and PVCs that do not respond to lidocaine or when lidocaine is contraindicated. For wide complex tachycardias that cannot be distinguished from VT, procainamide is considered an acceptable, potentially helpful intervention.[6] Procainamide is given by IV infusion.

Bretylium tosylate (Bretylol) is quite different from other antidysrhythmics. It causes a transient release of norepinephrine, after which it inhibits the release of norepinephrine and blocks the reuptake of norepinephrine, resulting in an increased fibrillatory threshold, prolonged effective refractory period, and suppression of reentry dysrhythmias. It is used for resistant VT and VF that does not respond to other therapy, such as defibrillation, epinephrine, and lidocaine.[6]

Beta-adrenergic blocking agents also have antidysrhythmic properties. They are useful in cardiac dysrhythmias caused by excessive sympathetic activity (paroxysmal atrial tachycardia, sinus tachycardia, and atrial fibrillation or flutter with rapid ventricular response). They also have been found to reduce the incidence of VF in post-MI patients who did not receive thrombolytic therapy.[6] The most important action of this group of drugs is to block sympathetic receptor sites in the myocardium (beta$_1$ receptors). Propranolol, atenolol, and metaprolol are examples of beta-adrenergic blocking agents. Although effective, these drugs can cause severe hypotension, bradycardia, and conduction delays. Therefore they are rarely used in prehospital care.

Adenosine (Adenocard) is a relatively new drug that is being used with increasing frequency in the prehospital setting.[5,17] Adenosine is an endogenous chemical present in all cells of the body. It slows conduction in the atrioventricular (AV) node and is effective in terminating supraventricular dysrhythmias caused by reentry. Adenosine is indicated for paroxysmal supraventricular tachycardias (PSVT), including those associated with Wolff-Parkinson-White syndrome. It is not useful for converting other supraventricular dysrhythmias that are unrelated to reentry, such as atrial fibrillation and atrial flutter. Current literature suggests that adenosine has a high success rate with minimal side effects.[5] Conversion dysrhythmias can occur, however, and at least two cases of serious adverse effects have been reported.[22]

Verapamil (Calan, Isoptin) is a calcium channel blocker used in the treatment of supraventricular dysrhythmias. Verapamil slows conduction in the AV node. Verapamil can cause severe hypotension and thus is rarely used in the prehospital setting. Verapamil should be used only in those patients with narrow complex PSVT or dysrhythmias known to be of supraventricular origin.[6] However, adenosine is currently the drug of choice for narrow complex PSVT initially. Because there is a higher incidence of recurrence of PSVT with adenosine than with verapamil, a sequence of the two drugs should be considered for persistent PSVT. Adenosine should be given twice, followed by verapamil twice if the patient's blood pressure has not dropped.

Catecholamines

Catecholamines are a group of structurally similar compounds that function as autonomic neurotransmitters. Three catecholamines are naturally occurring: epinephrine, norepinephrine, and dopamine. (These agents are also synthetically manufactured.) Epinephrine and norepinephrine are important neurotransmitters that influence normal neuronal and endocrine function. The role of dopamine in the autonomic nervous system is still not well understood. The fourth catecholamine, isoproterenol (Isuprel), is a synthetic drug.

Catecholamines act by directly stimulating adrenergic receptors and are referred to as sympathomimetic drugs. They produce a variety of physiologic effects. The actions of each catecholamine are determined by the specific receptor on which each acts (see Chapter 5). Each of the catecholamines has a specific role in ACLS.

Epinephrine (Adrenalin) is a critically important drug. It is useful in cardiac arrest (asystole, VF, pulseless VT, and PEA) because of its alpha-adrenergic stimulating properties. It is the first-line drug in each of these situations. What constitutes the most effective dose of epinephrine has been the focus of numerous studies. Historically, a standard adult dose of 1 mg given every 5 minutes has been used. The 1992 AHA guidelines recommend that this dosage continue to be used initially but repeated at 3- to 5-minute intervals. Higher doses should be considered only after the 1-mg dose has failed. If the initial dose of epinephrine does not elicit a favorable response, three different dosing regimens are considered acceptable, potentially helpful interventions.[6] The drug profile at the end of this chapter presents the various dosing regimens for adult and pediatric patients.

Dopamine (Intropin) is used primarily to improve blood pressure in the postresuscitation phase of cardiac arrest and in cardiogenic shock. Dopamine should not be used to raise blood pressure in hypovolemic patients unless fluid replacement has been accomplished. Doses ranging from 2 to 10 µg/kg/min stimulate beta-adrenergic receptors, resulting in improved cardiac output. At doses higher than 10 µg/kg/min, alpha-adrenergic receptor stimulation causes increased vasoconstriction.

Isoproterenol (Isuprel) is a beta-adrenergic agonist. It has potent inotropic and chronotropic properties that increase myocardial workload and can result in dysrhythmias and exacerbation of ischemia in patients with heart disease. The only indication for which isoproterenol is probably helpful is for refractory TDP and for immediate temporary control of hemodynamically significant bradycardia in heart transplant patients.[6] It should be used only with extreme caution in symptomatic bradycardia and is considered potentially helpful at low doses and potentially harmful at high doses.[6]

Norepinephrine (Levophed) has potent alpha-adrenergic and beta-adrenergic properties. ACLS guidelines suggest its use only for severe hypotension (systolic pressure less than 70). Once a systolic blood pressure of 70 to 100 is achieved, dopamine should be started. Norepinephrine is rarely administered in the field.

Anticholinergics

Anticholinergic drugs inhibit the action of acetylcholine. Anticholinergic drugs are also referred to as parasympatholytic agents. Atropine is the anticholinergic agent used most frequently in the prehospital setting. In cardiac emergencies it is the drug of choice for symptomatic bradycardias. It may also be beneficial in AV block and asystole.[5] In asystole it is given only after epinephrine has failed to elicit a response. The 1992

ACLS guidelines recommend a change in the time interval for administration from every 5 minutes to every 3 to 5 minutes. Atropine may be given intravenously or endotracheally. Specific doses are presented in the drug profile at the end of this chapter.

CONGESTIVE HEART FAILURE

Congestive heart failure (CHF) is a pathologic condition in which the damaged myocardium is unable to pump sufficient blood from the ventricles to provide adequate oxygenation for the body. There are many underlying causes of CHF, the most common being hypertension, MI, and pulmonary disease. Pulmonary edema is a severe form of CHF in which there is an accumulation of fluid in the lungs.

The patient in Case Presentation 3 typifies CHF. Her pulse was weak and thready, she was diaphoretic, and she had severe dyspnea. (There are noncardiac causes of pulmonary edema, but these occur far less frequently than those associated with CHF.)

The goals of treatment for CHF are: (1) to improve tissue oxygenation, (2) to improve myocardial contractility, and (3) to remove excess water and salt from the body to decrease the workload of the heart.

Drug therapy for pulmonary edema or CHF in the prehospital setting most often consists of the administration of high-flow oxygen, morphine sulfate, and a diuretic. Morphine is valuable because, in addition to its calming and sedative properties, it causes peripheral vasodilation that results in decreased venous return to the heart (see drug profile on page 260).

Reduction of excess water and sodium is accomplished through the use of diuretics. Although there are numerous diuretics available, two are of particular value in emergency medicine: furosemide (Lasix) and bumetanide Bumex). Both drugs are loop diuretics and have similar actions. Bumetanide is more expensive, however, and offers no apparent advantage over furosemide for prehospital use. Thus furosemide is the most commonly used diuretic in the field. Furosemide causes diuresis and decreased venous return to the heart, making it valuable in the management of acute pulmonary edema and CHF.

Other drugs that can be used in CHF are nitroglycerin and dobutamine (Dobutrex). Nitroglycerin's vasodilating properties reduce venous return and, thus, myocardial workload. Dobutamine is a synthetic sympathomimetic drug that is structurally similar to dopamine, with potent inotropic properties. It is useful in the treatment of CHF but is used infrequently in the field.

Case Presentation 3 demonstrates appropriate interventions for CHF. The first priority is high-flow oxygen to increase the concentration of arterial oxygen. Drugs that improve myocardial contractility are not usually given until the patient reaches the hospital. Furosemide and morphine helped to reduce venous return, myocardial workload, and dyspnea in the patient in this case.

HYPERTENSION

Hypertension is generally defined as systolic blood pressure greater than 140 mm Hg and/or a diastolic blood pressure greater than 90 mm Hg. Frequently, people with hypertension are asymptomatic until secondary complications, such as stroke, coronary artery disease, or renal failure, appear.

True hypertensive emergencies are less easily defined. Blood pressure may be extremely elevated in some cases, whereas in others it is only moderately high. The critical component in identifying hypertensive emergencies is the occurrence of symptoms (e.g., headache, blurred vision, confusion, stupor, seizure, and possibly coma) in the presence of a high diastolic pressure. In these situations it is important to achieve an immediate decrease in blood pressure.

The specific agents used to treat hypertension vary with local protocols. Those that have been used in the prehospital setting include diazoxide, hydralazine, and nitroprusside. These agents bring about a prompt reduction in arterial blood pressure and can result in severe hypotension. Thus it is preferable that their administration be deferred until the patient reaches the hospital if possible. These agents are used less frequently than nifedipine.

Nifedipine (Adalat, Procardia), a calcium channel blocker, has become the drug of choice for the prehospital management of hypertensive emergencies. Its primary action is the relaxation of vascular smooth muscle resulting in vasodilation, thereby reducing peripheral vascular resistance. It is given sublingually.

When hypertension is associated with MI, nitroglycerin may be helpful in reducing arterial pressure. In these situations nifedipine may be harmful because it has a negative inotropic effect.

SUMMARY

Cardiovascular emergencies are among the most common emergencies confronting paramedics. Patients can present with a variety of signs and symptoms ranging from chest pain and dyspnea to complete cardiac arrest. Drug therapy is a key component of patient management.

The management of chest pain includes the administration of oxygen, nitroglycerin, nitrous oxide, and morphine sulfate. Life-threatening dysrhythmias require timely recognition and appropriate intervention. Lidocaine is the drug used most frequently for ventricular dysrhythmias, but other antidysrhythmics are available to paramedics. It is important that paramedics understand the action and indications of each of the antidysrhythmics used in the prehospital setting.

Patients with CHF and hypertension can benefit also from prehospital drug therapy. Oxygen therapy and diuretics are the mainstay of the prehospital management of CHF. Hypertensive emergencies are less common but require immediate intervention. The drug of choice for hypertensive emergencies in the prehospital setting is nifedipine.

The medications discussed in this chapter must be used in conjunction with other interventions as appropriate. Paramedics must adequately assess the patient's condition and consider the best form of management. Paramedics should be acutely aware of local protocols as well as AHA guidelines.

REFERENCES

1. Auf der heide T: Prehospital bicarbonate use in cardiac arrest, *Amer J Emerg Med* 10:4, 1992.
2. Chameides LE: *Textbook of pediatric advanced life support*, 1990, American Heart Association.
3. Cherry RA: PALS: managing the critically ill child, *Prehosp Care Rep* 1(6):43, 1991.
4. Dicksinson ET: Magnesium comes of age, *J Emerg Med Serv* 17(4):60, 1992.
5. Duffy SP, Murphy PM, Shatzle JC: Adenosine—an old drug learns new trick, *J Emerg Med Serv* 17(4):58, 1990.
6. Emergency Cardiac Care Committee and Subcommittees, *American Heart Association guidelines for cardiopulmonary resuscitation and emergency cardiac care, III: Pediatric Advanced Life Support*, JAMA 268:2199, 1992.
7. Emergency Cardiac Care Committee and Subcommittees, *American Heart Association guidelines for cardiopulmonary resuscitation and emergency cardiac care, IV: Pediatric Advanced Life Support*, JAMA 268:2262, 1992.
8. Foley JJ: Drug update deltiagem IV (cardigem) for atrial fibrillation and flutter, *J Emerg Nurs* 18(4):343, 1992.
9. Garza MA: Inside EMS—new study casts doubt on equality of two thrombolytic drugs, *J Emerg Med Serv* 16(1):21, 1991.
10. Gleeson B: Loosening the grip of anginal pain, *Nurs 91* 21(1):41, 1991.
11. Goetting MG, Paradis NA: High-dose epinephrine improves outcome from pediatric cardiac arrest, *Ann Emerg Med* 20:22, 1991.
12. Handberg E, Kieth T, Rucinski P: Clot busters—the future of EMS thrombolytics, *J Emerg Med Serv* 17(4):74, 1992.

13. Kereiakes DJ et al: Time delays in the diagnosis and treatment of acute myocardial infarction: a tale of eight cities, *Amer Heart J* 120:773, 1990.
14. MacPhail E, editor: The role of heparin and aspirin during thrombolytic intervention in acute myocardial infarction, *Heartbeat* 1(3):1, 1990.
15. MacPhail E: Transport considerations for a patient receiving t-PA, *Heartbeat* 1(4):5, 1990.
16. MacPhail E, Searle L, editors: Thrombolysis and patient safety, *Heartbeat* 2(2):1, 1991.
17. McCabe JL et al: Intravenous adenosine in the prehospital treatment of paroxysmal supraventricular tachycardia, *Ann Emerg Med* 21(4):358, 1992.
18. Merlin M, Janeria LF: TdP: an irregular rhythm, *Emerg* 22(5):18, 1990.
19. Newman M, editor: Jury still out on high-dose epinephrine, *Curr Emerg Card Care* 2(2):1, 1991.
20. Ornata LJ: High-dose epinephrine during resuscitation: a word of caution, *JAMA* 265(9):1160, 1991.
21. Perkin RM: Facts and dilemmas resuscitating pediatric cardiac arrest victims, *J Emerg Med Serv* 17(6):68, 1992.
22. Reed R, Falk JL, O'Brien J: Untoward reaction to adenosine therapy for supraventricular tachycardia, *Amer J Emerg Med* 9(6):556, 1991.
23. Rottman SJ, Larmon Baxter: Nitroglycerine lingual aerosol in prehospital emergency care, *Prehosp Disast Med* 4(3):11, 1989.
24. Schneider SM et al: Endotracheal versus intravenous epinephrine in the prehospital treatment of cardiac arrest, *Prehosp Disast Med* 5(4):341, 1990.
25. Teplitz L: Clinical close-up on lidocaine, *Nurs* 19(9):44, 1989.
26. *Textbook of advanced cardiac life support*, ed 2, American Heart Association, 45 and 97, 1987.
27. Varshavsky SY: Prehospital thrombolysis in acute myocardial infarction, *Prehosp Disast Med* 7(1):57, 1992.
28. Wilson V: Action stat! Complications of thrombolytic therapy, *Nurs 91* 21(1):41, 1991.

DRUG PROFILES
◆ Adenosine (Adenocard)

Adenosine is a new and exciting breakthrough in the treatment of supraventricular tachycardia. It is an endogenous chemical that is found in all cells of the body. It is unrelated to all other antidysrhythmic agents.

Mechanism of action

Adenosine slows conduction time through the AV node. It has proven useful in blocking reentry pathways through the AV node in supraventricular tachydysrhythmias that have been previously resistant to other antidysrhythmic drugs.

Indications

Adenosine is indicated only in the treatment of PSVTs, including those associated with Wolff-Parkinson-White syndrome. It is not effective in converting rhythms other than PSVT, such as atrial fibrillation and ventricular tachycardia.

Contraindications

- second- or third-degree block
- sick sinus syndrome
- dysrhythmias other than PSVT

Precautions

Adenosine can produce bronchoconstriction in patients with asthma. This problem must be anticipated in the field, particularly when there is no source of medical history.

Side effects

Because the half-life of adenosine is less than 10 seconds, side effects are usually transient. At the time the dysrhythmia is interrupted, several new dysrhythmias may appear temporarily. PVCs, premature atrial contractions, sinus tachycardia, sinus bradycardia, and AV block are frequently seen prior to conversion to normal sinus rhythm. These conversion dysrhythmias are typically short-lived and seldom require intervention. One study reports two cases with significant side effects, prolonged sinus arrest with syncope and syncope with prolonged bradycardia and hypotension.[5] Other side effects include:
- facial flushing
- headache
- shortness of breath

- dizziness, light-headedness
- nausea
- chest pain

Interactions

Potential additive interactions exist when administered to patients who are on other medications that slow AV conduction (e.g., digoxin, calcium channel blockers). Methylxanthines (e.g., caffeines, theophylline preparations) antagonize the effects of adenosine which may require an increase in dose. In some cases the antagonistic effect of methylxanthines has rendered the dose of adenosine completely ineffective.

Dosage

Adults: initial dose of adenosine is 6 mg rapid IV bolus; if dysrhythmias fail to convert within 1 to 2 minutes, dosage should be increased to 12 mg and repeated; after 2 minutes, 12-mg dose may be given a second time, if necessary.

Infants and children: initial dose of 0.1 mg/kg; if no effect the dose may be doubled. The maximum single dose of adenosine should not exceed 12 mg.

Administration

Adenosine is administered by rapid IV bolus, over a 1- to 2-second period. The emphasis here is on *rapid* administration, which is imperative because of the extremely short half-life of the drug. The drug should be injected as proximal to the heart as possible and followed by a rapid flush of fluid, such as normal saline. The antecubital veins are preferable to the veins of the hands and forearm.

◆ Alteplase Recombinant (Activase)

Alteplase is a tPA that is produced by recombinant DNA technology.

Mechanism of action

Alteplase binds to fibrin in a thrombus (clot) and converts the entrapped plasminogen to plasmin. This results in local fibrinolysis (the dissolution of fibrin clots). The dissolution of coronary thrombi may limit infarct size.

Indications

The only indication for alteplase in the prehospital setting is acute MI (within 4 to 6 hours of onset).

Contraindications

Because thrombolytic therapy increases risk of bleeding, administration is contraindicated in the following situations:
- recent cerebrovascular accident (within 2 months)
- recent intracranial or intraspinal surgery or trauma (within 2 months)
- intracranial neoplasm
- AV malformation or aneurysm
- bleeding disorders
- severe uncontrolled hypertension

In the following situations extreme caution should be used, with the potential therapeutic outcome weighed against the risk of administration:
- pregnancy
- age greater than 75 years
- recent gastrointestinal or genitourinary bleeding (within 10 days)
- recent trauma (within 10 days)
- pericarditis, endocarditis
- liver dysfunction
- recent surgery (within 10 days)

Precautions

Reperfusion dysrhythmias are a frequent phenomenon associated with thrombolytic therapy. These dysrhythmias (sinus bradycardia, accelerated idioventricular rhythm, PVCs, and VT) are no different from those usually seen with acute MI, and standard therapy should be used. Drugs to treat bradycardia and ventricular irritability should be immediately available at the time thrombolytic therapy is initiated. Some protocols call for the use of prophylactic lidocaine. Because of the increased risk of bleeding, invasive procedures should be avoided if possible. IVs are usually started with catheters not larger than an 18 gauge.

Side effects

- bleeding
- fever
- reperfusion dysrhythmias
- transient ischemic attacks
- phlebitis at IV site

Note: Despite the risk of bleeding that exists, cases of serious hemorrhage are rare.

Interactions

The interaction of cardioactive drugs with alteplase has not been studied. Drugs that alter platelet function, such as aspirin, may increase bleeding if administered prior to, during, or after alteplase administration.

Dosage

Adults: (weighing 60 kg or more)—a total dose of 100 mg
        (weighing less than 60 kg)—1.25 mg/kg
Infants and children: Not recommended for pediatric patients.

Administration

Different protocols exist across the country for administration of thrombolytic agents in the prehospital setting. The manufacturer recommends the following for patients weighing 60 kg or more: (1) 60 mg given over the first hour with the initial 6 to 10 mg being administered over 1 to 2 minutes by IV bolus and the remainder of the dose by IV infusion, (2) 20 mg given over the second hour, and (3) 20 mg given over the third hour. For patients weighing less than 60 kg: (1) 0.75 mg/kg given over the first hour with the initial 0.075 to 0.125 mg/kg being administered over 1 to 2 minutes by IV bolus and the remainder of the dose by IV infusion, (2) 0.25 mg/kg given over the second hour, and (3) 0.25 mg/kg given over the third hour. Many protocols include the concomitant use of heparin to maintain anticoagulation.

◆ Atropine Sulfate

Atropine sulfate is an anticholinergic (parasympatholytic) drug.

Mechanism of action

Atropine produces its action by blocking the effects of acetylcholine at muscarinic receptors. Atropine causes dilation of the pupils (mydriasis), paralysis of the ciliary muscle (cycloplegia), central nervous system excitation, relaxation of the bronchioles, urinary retention, decreased motility of the gastrointestinal tract, and increased heart rate. (Stimulation of muscarinic receptors causes a decrease in heart rate; thus, blockade of these receptors by a muscarinic antagonist, such as atropine, increases heart rate.)

Indications

- used for the management of symptomatic bradycardias
- indicated in asystole when epinephrine has not been effective
- used in poisonings by certain mushrooms, insecticides, and nerve gas

Contraindications

Atropine is contraindicated in patients with glaucoma or myasthenia gravis.

Precautions

Atropine can cause tachycardia and should be administered cautiously in patients with MI or myocardial ischemia. Excessive doses can cause delirium or coma. Ventricular tachycardia and ventricular fibrillation have occurred with atropine administration.

Side effects

- dry mouth
- blurred vision
- urinary retention
- constipation
- tachycardia

Interactions

Antihistamines, phenothiazine antipsychotics, and tricyclic antidepressants enhance the effects of atropine.

Dosage

Adults: For symptomatic bradycardias—0.5- to 1.0-mg IV push; dose may be repeated every 3 to 5 minutes up to a maximum dose of 0.04 mg/kg; 3 mg (0.04 mg/kg) results in full vagal blockade.[6] Doses of less than 0.5 mg may cause a further slowing of heart rate. In asystole and PEA—initial dose of 1.0 mg; may be repeated in 3 to 5 minutes.[6]

In poisonings—larger doses are required; usually initial dose of 2.0 mg (use of atropine in poisonings is discussed in Chapter 14).

Infants and children: 0.02 mg/kg (minimal dose of 0.1 mg and a maximum dose of 0.5 mg in child, and 1.0 mg in adolescent).[7]

Administration

In the emergency setting atropine is administered via IV push. It is available in a prefilled syringe containing 0.5 mg in 5 ml of solution. In the absence of IV access, atropine can be administered via an endotracheal tube or an intraosseous line.

The paramedic should be careful to avoid accidental exposure of the eye when preparing and administering injections of atropine. Atropine causes paralysis of the ciliary muscle, resulting in blurred vision.

◆ Bretylium Tosylate (Bretylol)

Bretylium tosylate is quite different from all the other antidysrhythmics discussed. It does not suppress automaticity and has no effect on conduction velocity.

Mechanism of action

Bretylium causes an initial but transient release of norepinephrine. This

effect lasts approximately 20 minutes. Bretylium then inhibits the release of norepinephrine and blocks the reuptake of norepinephrine, resulting in the depletion of norepinephrine. This action results in:
- increase of the fibrillation threshold in the ventricles
- prolonged effective refractory period
- suppression of reentry dysrhythmias

Indications

Bretylium is indicated in the treatment of VT and VF that are refractory to lidocaine and defibrillation, recurrent VF despite the use of epinephrine and lidocaine, VT (with a pulse) that fails to respond to lidocaine or procainamide, and wide-complex tachycardias not controlled by lidocaine and adenosine.[6]

Contraindications

There are no contraindications when used for the treatment of life-threatening dysrhythmias (VT and VF). It is contraindicated in torsades de pointes.

Precautions

Bretylium can result in prolonged hypotension in the postresuscitation phase of treatment.

Side effects

A frequently observed side effect with bretylium administration is an initial, transient elevation in blood pressure followed by hypotension. Other side effects include:
- dizziness, syncope
- angina
- bradycardia
- nasal stuffiness
- when administered by rapid IV injection in the conscious patient, can produce nausea and vomiting

Interactions

Bretylium may have additive or antagonistic effects when used concurrently with other antidysrhythmics.

Dosage

Adults: For VF—5 mg/kg IV; if no response, increase to 10 mg/kg and repeat at 5-minute intervals not to exceed 30 to 35 mg/kg every 24 hours.[6] For other ventricular dysrhythmias—5 to 10 mg/kg over a period of 8 to 10 minutes.

Children: No published data is available for use in pediatrics. For VF that does not respond to defibrillation and epinephrine, the AHA guidelines recommend the same initial dose as for adults (5 mg/kg). If ineffective, an additional dose of 10 mg/kg can be administered.[7]

Administration

For use in VF, bretylium may be administered by rapid IV push over a period of 15 to 30 seconds. To prevent nausea and vomiting in the conscious patient it is best diluted and given by infusion over a longer period of time (10 to 30 minutes). It should be noted that bretylium is most effective in the conversion of VF when followed immediately by defibrillation. Following successful dysrhythmia conversion with IV bolus therapy, a maintenance infusion of bretylium should be initiated and administered at a rate of 1 to 2 mg/min.

◆ Dobutamine (Dobutrex)

Dobutamine is a synthetic sympathomimetic drug.

Mechanism of action

At low doses dobutamine acts selectively on beta$_1$-adrenergic receptors to increase contractility with little effect on heart rate. Dobutamine does not cause the release of endogenous norepinephrine. At higher doses dobutamine increases heart rate and conduction velocity and stimulates beta$_2$-adrenergic receptors, resulting in vasodilation. The hemodynamic effect of dobutamine is to increase cardiac output and to decrease peripheral vascular resistance.

Indications

Dobutamine is indicated in CHF and in hemodynamically significant right ventricular infarction.

Contraindications

• tachydysrhythmias
• severe hypotension

Precautions

Dobutamine should be used with caution in patients with recent MI.

Side effects

• dysrhythmias

- headache
- nausea
- tremor

Interactions

The effects of beta-adrenergic blockers and some of the antihypertensive agents may be blocked by dobutamine.

Dosage

Like dopamine, the dosage of dobutamine is titrated to the patient's hemodynamic response with the smallest effective dose being used. In some patients very low doses (0.5 µg/kg/min) may be effective. The usual dose range is 2.5 to 20.0 µg/kg/min in pediatric and adult patients.

Administration

Dobutamine has a very short half-life (about 2 minutes) and must be administered by IV infusion. Usually two ampules (500 mg per ampule) are mixed in 250 ml of D₅W, resulting in a concentration of 4 mg/ml. The increased heart rate and blood pressure fluctuation that is seen with higher doses of dobutamine can result in myocardial ischemia. Patients need to be monitored closely for signs of ischemia, such as chest pain or dysrhythmias.

◆ Dopamine (Intropin)

Dopamine is a naturally occurring catecholamine that is the physiologic precursor of norepinephrine. Because it does not increase heart rate or myocardial oxygen consumption to the extent that epinephrine and isoproterenol do, it is the preferred drug for hypotension associated with cardiogenic shock and CHF.

Mechanism of action

Dopamine acts directly on dopaminergic, alpha- and beta-adrenergic receptors. Its action, like that of epinephrine, is dose-related. At low doses (1 to 2 µg/kg/min), dopaminergic receptors are stimulated, resulting in vasodilation of renal, mesenteric, and cerebral arteries. With doses ranging from 2 to 10 µg/kg/min, beta stimulation results in increased cardiac output with minimal changes in systemic vascular resistance or preload.

Alpha adrenergic effects predominate with doses greater than 10 µg/kg/min, causing vasoconstriction in the renal, mesenteric, and peripheral arteries and veins. At doses greater than 20 µg/kg/min the effects of dopamine are similar to those of norepinephrine.

Indications

- used to improve cardiac output and blood pressure in shock states; treatment of choice in cardiogenic shock; in hypovolemic shock, volume replacement must be accomplished prior to using dopamine.
- congestive heart failure

Contraindications

Administration to women receiving oxytocin may result in severe persistent hypertension.

Precautions

Dopamine is the most widely used drug for the treatment of shock. Dopamine increases heart rate and can cause or exacerbate both supraventricular and ventricular dysrhythmias. Reduction in the rate of infusion or discontinuance of the infusion may be necessary.

Although dopamine does not increase myocardial workload to the same extent as epinephrine, norepinephrine, and isoproterenol, it can increase myocardial oxygen consumption without significant improvement in coronary blood flow. In some patients cardiac status may worsen with the administration of dopamine. Careful attention must be given to continual assessment of the patient receiving dopamine.

Side effects

- dysrhythmias
- hypertension
- headache
- nausea and vomiting

Interactions

- Tricyclic antidepressants potentiate the effects of dopamine.
- Patients receiving monoamine oxidase inhibitors require a reduced dose of dopamine.
- Dopamine may not be stable in alkaline solutions and should not be given in the same IV line with sodium bicarbonate.[6]
- Pink or brown solutions indicate expiration and should not be used.

Dosage

The dose that improves cardiac output (beta stimulation) with only moderate increases in peripheral vascular resistance (alpha stimulation) is 2 to 10 µg/kg/min.

The initial rate of infusion is 2 to 5 µg/kg/min. Higher doses may be required to achieve an adequate blood pressure in some patients. The maximum dose is 50 µg/kg/min. However, doses generally do not exceed 20 µg/kg/min.

Administration

Because dopamine is rapidly inactivated, it must be given by continuous IV infusion. Dopamine can cause tissue necrosis and sloughing. Care should be taken to prevent infiltration or leakage at the infusion site. A central line is preferable for administration.

When central access is not feasible, the large veins of the arm should be used. The small veins of the hand and forearm should be avoided. Patient response to dopamine varies. It is therefore titrated to the patient's hemodynamic response. Usually one to two ampules containing 200 mg of the drug are diluted in 250 ml of D_5W.

◆ Epinephrine (Adrenalin)

Epinephrine is a direct-acting catecholamine secreted by the adrenal medulla in response to sympathetic stimulation. Epinephrine is used in prehospital medicine for respiratory emergencies and anaphylactic reactions (see Chapter 7), and cardiac emergencies.

Mechanism of action

Epinephrine stimulates $beta_1$, $beta_2$, and $alpha_1$ receptors. Its effect on beta receptors is significantly more profound than its effect on alpha receptors. $Beta_1$ stimulation results in increased force of contraction, increased heart rate, and increased AV conduction. Epinephrine can cause spontaneous firing of Purkinje fibers and has been shown to initiate spontaneous myocardial contraction in asystole. In VF or pulseless VT, epinephrine is known to increase the likelihood of successful defibrillation. $Beta_2$ stimulation results in bronchodilation and vasodilation of the vessels in skeletal muscle. Stimulation of the $alpha_1$ receptors causes vasoconstriction.

The vascular effects of epinephrine are dose-related. At low doses $beta_2$ receptors predominate with a decrease in total peripheral resistance and a decrease in blood pressure. With larger doses alpha effects predominate with an increase in peripheral vascular resistance and an increase in blood pressure. The increased vasoconstriction and increased perfusion pressure resulting from epinephrine's stimulation of alpha receptors are desirable in cardiac arrest.

Indications

- asystole, VF, pulseless VT, and PEA
- acute bronchospasm associated with asthma or COPD
- anaphylaxis

Contraindications

There are no contraindications for the use of epinephrine in cardiac arrest.

Precautions

- Epinephrine should be protected from light.
- Epinephrine is unstable in alkaline solutions, such as sodium bicarbonate.
- Pink or brown solutions should not be used, as they indicate expiration.

Side effects

- central nervous system stimulation results in fear and anxiety
- headache, dizziness, pallor
- nausea and vomiting
- palpitations

Interactions

Monoamine oxidase inhibitors and tricyclic antidepressants intensify and prolong epinephrine's effects. Beta$_1$-adrenergic blocking agents can reduce the side effects of epinephrine, such as dysrhythmias and chest pain. These interactions, although important, should not prevent the use of epinephrine in cardiac arrest.

Dosage

Adults: In cardiac arrest: the recommended dose of epinephrine is 1 mg (10 ml of a 1:10,000 solution) in adults administered IV every 3 to 5 minutes. Higher doses of epinephrine are an acceptable, potentially helpful intervention and should be considered only after the 1 mg dose has failed.[6] Regimens for intermediate, escalating, and high doses are found in the algorithms for VT, VF, PEA, and asystole in Appendix A.

For endotracheal administration: a dose at least 2 to 2.5 times the peripheral IV dose may be needed.

For acute bronchospasm associated with asthma and COPD: the dose is 0.3 mg to 0.5 mg (0.3 ml to 0.5 ml of a 1:1000 solution) subcutaneously. The dose may be repeated every 5 to 20 minutes to a total of three doses.

Children: For bradycardia: the recommended dose is 0.01 mg/kg (0.1 ml/kg of a 1:10,000 solution) intravenously or intraosseously. If the endotracheal route is used, the dose should be increased to 0.1 mg/kg (0.1 ml/kg of a 1:1000 solution).

In cardiac arrest: the initial dose of epinephrine is 0.01 mg/kg (0.1 ml/kg of a 1:10,000 solution. Second and subsequent doses should be

0.1 mg/kg (0.1 ml of a 1:1000) solution. The second dose should be administered within 3 to 5 minutes of the first dose and every 3 to 5 minutes thereafter.[7] Second and subsequent doses as high as 0.2 mg/kg (0.2 ml/kg of a 1:1000 solution) may be helpful.

For asthma: the dose is 0.01 mg/kg (0.01 ml/kg of a 1:1000) solution given subcutaneously. The dose may be repeated every 5 to 20 minutes for a total of three doses.

Administration

In cardiac arrest, epinephrine should be administered intravenously. In the absence of IV access, epinephrine can be administered endotracheally.

Endotracheal administration of epinephrine has become commonplace. A recent study, however, suggests that initial treatment with endotracheal epinephrine is less effective than IV administration of epinephrine in restoring a pulse in out-of-hospital cardiac arrest victims and that the endotracheal route should be reserved for patients without IV access.[24]

◆ Furosemide (Lasix)

Furosemide is a loop diuretic given for its diuretic and antihypertensive properties.

Mechanism of action

Furosemide is a potent diuretic that inhibits the reabsorption of sodium and chloride in the kidneys. It increases renal excretion of water, sodium, chloride, magnesium, and calcium. Furosemide also causes venodilation, which reduces venous return to the heart. Its onset of action is about 5 minutes with IV administration.

Indications

- pulmonary and peripheral edema
- CHF
- hypertension

Contraindications

- pregnancy and lactation
- hypovolemia
- hypokalemia

Precautions

Furosemide should be used cautiously in liver disease, electrolyte depletion, and anuria.

Side effects

- when given rapidly, or in doses several times higher than the usual dose, furosemide can cause transient deafness
- hypokalemia
- hyperglycemia
- hyperuricemia
- weakness, dizziness
- hypotension

Interactions

Additive interactions are possible with antihypertensives, nitrates, and other diuretics.

Dosage

Adults and children: 0.5 to 1.0 mg/kg, slow IV push or intramuscularly

Administration

Furosemide should be administered by IV push in the prehospital setting. In the absence of IV access it may be administered intramuscularly.

◆ Isoproterenol (Isuprel)

Isoproterenol is a synthetic catecholamine that acts exclusively on beta-adrenergic receptors.

Mechanism of action

Isoproterenol stimulates beta-adrenergic receptors. It has potent, positive inotropic and chronotropic properties, resulting in increased cardiac output despite its vasodilatory effect. This increase in cardiac output is accompanied by marked increases in myocardial oxygen consumption that can exacerbate or lead to myocardial ischemia. Isoproterenol has therefore been replaced by other inotropic agents that are less likely to increase myocardial oxygen demand.

Indications

Isoproterenol is indicated in refractory torsades de pointes and temporary control of hemodynamically significant bradycardias in heart transplant patients. Isoproterenol should be used with extreme caution, if at all, for symptomatic bradycardias.[6]

Contraindications

- pulseless ventricular tachycardia; ventricular ectopy; tachydysrhythmias

- VF
- PEA
- asystole

Precautions

Isoproterenol should be given cautiously in patients with ischemic heart disease.

Side effects

- dysrhythmias
- palpitations
- hypotension
- angina
- headache
- flushing

Interactions

- As with the other catecholamines, monoamine oxidase inhibitors and tricyclic antidepressants potentiate the effect of isoproterenol.
- Patients taking digitalis should not receive isoproterenol.

Dosage

The starting dose is 1 to 2 µg/min with gradual increases in infusion rate until a heart rate of 60 beats/min or a systolic blood pressure of 90 mm Hg is achieved. The infusion rate should not exceed 10 µg/min. Isoproterenol is not recommended for use in children in the field.

Administration

Isoproterenol is administered by IV infusion. One ampule containing 1 mg of the drug is diluted in 500 ml of D_5W to yield a concentration of 2 µg/ml.

◆ Lidocaine hydrochloride

Lidocaine is the antidysrhythmic agent used most frequently in the prehospital setting.

Mechanism of action

Lidocaine decreases ventricular automaticity and excitability and raises the fibrillation threshold. It decreases conduction in ischemic cardiac tissue without adversely affecting normal conduction.[25] Lidocaine has little effect on myocardial contractility.

Indications

Lidocaine is the drug of choice in the treatment of ventricular dysrhythmias, including VT, VF, and malignant PVCs. Because lidocaine exerts little effect on the AV node and atrial myocardium, it is of little or no use in the treatment of supraventricular dysrhythmias.

Contraindications

- advanced AV block (Mobitz II and third-degree blocks)
- torsades de pointes

Precautions

Caution should be used when administering lidocaine to patients with heart rates lower than 60 or with a history of liver disease.

Side effects

- drowsiness
- dizziness
- confusion
- hypotension
- nausea, vomiting
- dysrhythmias
- respiratory depression
- cardiac arrest

Interactions

Lidocaine causes additive cardiac depression and toxicity when given in combination with other Class I antidysrhythmics (phenytoin, procainamide, quinidine, and propranolol).

Dosage

Adults: Initial bolus of 1 to 1.5 mg/kg; additional doses of 0.5 to 1.5 mg/kg may be repeated at 3- to 5-minute intervals to a total dose of 3 mg/kg. The more aggressive dosing regimen is recommended in cardiac arrest. If defibrillation and epinephrine fail to convert VF, the 1.5 mg bolus should be used.[6] After perfusion is reestablished, a continuous infusion should be initiated at a rate of 2 to 4 mg/min. Patients over the age of 70 or with decreased cardiac output or hepatic dysfunction should receive a decreased dose. These patients should be given the normal bolus dose first, followed by half the normal maintenance infusion.[6]

Children: 1 mg/kg bolus as loading dose, followed by continuous infusion of 20 to 50 μg/kg/min.

Administration

Lidocaine is administered via the IV route. The initial dose is given by IV bolus. Following conversion, a maintenance infusion is administered at 2 to 4 mg/min and titrated according to the patient's response. The maintenance infusion is usually prepared by diluting 1 g lidocaine in 250 or 500 ml D_5W to yield 2 to 4 mg/ml. A solution containing 2 mg/ml is referred as a 2:1 lidocaine solution. A solution containing 4 mg/ml is referred to as a 4:1 lidocaine solution.

◆ Nifedipine (Adalat, Procardia)

Nifedipine is a calcium channel blocker.

Mechanism of action

Nifedipine acts to block slow calcium channels, resulting in the dilatation of systemic and coronary arteries. It decreases arterial blood pressure, preload, afterload, and myocardial oxygen consumption.

Indications

The major indication of nifedipine in the prehospital setting is hypertensive crises. It can be used for angina.

Contraindications

- hypotension
- hypovolemia

Precautions

Caution should be used in administering nifedipine to patients with CHF.

Side effects

- headache
- dizziness
- hypotension
- syncope
- reflex tachycardia

Interactions

Severe hypotension or congestive heart failure can occur if used with beta-adrenergic blockers.

Dosage

Adults: 5 to 10 mg sublingually; dose may be repeated every 30 to 60 minutes. Children: Not recommended for prehospital use.

Administration

Nifedipine is available in a capsule. The capsule is pierced and the liquid squirted under the tongue, or the patient is asked to chew the capsule and hold the liquid in his or her mouth for several seconds prior to swallowing.

◆ Nitroglycerin

Nitroglycerin is an antianginal agent that belongs to a group of drugs referred to as nitrates.

Mechanism of action

Nitroglycerin relaxes vascular smooth muscle, resulting in peripheral vasodilation. The resulting decrease in peripheral vascular resistance decreases myocardial workload and myocardial oxygen demand.

Indications

Relief of acute anginal pain.

Contraindications

- head trauma or cerebral hemorrhage
- hypotension
- hypovolemia

Precautions

Nitroglycerin should also be used with great caution in glaucoma, as it may increase intraocular pressure.

Side effects

- vasodilation results in headache
- hypotension
- nausea and vomiting
- tachycardia
- skin rash

Interactions

- alcohol–when combined with nitroglycerin, may cause severe hypotension
- aspirin–interaction results in increased serum nitrate concentrations
- calcium channel blockers–additive interaction can result in symptomatic orthostatic hypotension

Dosage

Adults: 0.3 to 0.4 mg
Children: Not recommended for prehospital use in children.

Administration

One sublingual tablet or one lingual aerosol metered-dose spray should be administered as soon as possible after the onset of chest pain. Doses may be repeated every 3 to 5 minutes as needed, up to three doses. If relief is not obtained, medical direction or local protocols should be consulted for additional orders, usually involving morphine sulfate administration. Patients should be instructed to remain in a recumbent position to decrease the effects of hypotension.

Sublingual tablets: If the patient has never taken sublingual nitroglycerin, explain that there will be a fizzing sensation and that the tablet should be allowed to dissolve completely under the tongue without swallowing it.

Lingual aerosol spray: Do not shake the can when administering. The can should be held vertically when spraying under the patient's tongue. The patient should be instructed not to inhale the liquid and to refrain from swallowing for several seconds.

Nitroglycerin preparations should be stored in a cool environment away from bright sunlight. The expiration date should be checked frequently, as these preparations generally do not have a long shelf life.

◆ **Procainamide Hydrochloride (Pronestyl)**

Procainamide is an antidysrhythmic that is generally regarded as a cardiac depressant. Although lidocaine is the antidysrhythmic of choice, procainamide is useful in treating ventricular dysrhythmias that do not respond to lidocaine or for treating patients who have a known history of allergy to lidocaine.

Mechanism of action

Procainamide decreases cardiac excitability and automaticity and slows conduction velocity. In the damaged heart it can decrease contractility, thereby leading to decreased cardiac output and hypotension.

Indications

Procainamide is primarily used for PVCs or recurrent VTs that do not respond to lidocaine. It is also used for supraventricular dysrhythmias, including atrial premature contractions, paroxysmal atrial tachycardia, and atrial fibrillation. It can be used for wide-complex tachydysrhythmias that cannot be distinguished from VT, but it is not the first-line drug of choice.

Contraindications

- AV block
- bradycardia

- torsades de pointes
- tricyclic antidepressant poisoning

Precautions

Procainamide should be used with great caution in cases of myocardial infarction, CHF, digitalis toxicity, and hepatic and renal dysfunction.

Side effects

The most serious side effects of procainamide administration are associated with the drug's depressant action on the myocardium. These include:
- bradycardia
- hypotension
- heart block
- dysrhythmias
- conduction delays (prolonged PR interval, prolonged QT interval, or widened QRS)

Other side effects include skin rash, nausea, vomiting, confusion, and dizziness.

Interactions

Procainamide can have either an additive or an antagonistic effect when combined with other antidysrhythmics. Additive effects occur when given in combination with drugs that have anticholinergic properties, such as many antidepressants, atropine, antihistamines, and haloperidol.

Dosage

Adults: 20 mg/min by IV infusion (up to a total dose of 17 mg/kg).
Children: Because of the seriousness of potential side effects Procainamide is not usually used for children in the prehospital setting.

Administration

Procainamide is administered by IV infusion at a rate of 20 mg/min until the dysrhythmia terminates, hypotension ensues, the width of the QRS increases by half, or a total of 17 mg/kg has been given.[6] The drug should be protected from light and the solution inspected prior to giving the dose. It should be clear to pale yellow and should be discarded when discoloration is noted. The patient's ECG and blood pressure should be monitored continuously while receiving IV procainamide. Because of the seriousness of potential side effects with IV administration, IV use should be discontinued when the cardiac dysrhythmias are suppressed or hypotension occurs. Progression of side effects should be reported to medical direction immediately. In light of possible serious interaction with many other drugs, every effort should be made to ascertain currently prescribed drug therapy and use of over-the-counter drugs.

◆ Sodium Bicarbonate

Sodium bicarbonate is an alkalinizing agent.

Mechanism of action

Sodium bicarbonate neutralizes excess acid.

Indications

Sodium bicarbonate is indicated in metabolic acidosis. It is not routinely used in cardiac arrest and may worsen outcome when used. Metabolic acidosis is best managed by adequate ventilation and oxygenation. Sodium bicarbonate is beneficial in patients with preexisting metabolic acidosis, hyperkalemia, or tricyclic antidepressant or phenobarbital overdose.[6] Sodium bicarbonate is best administered on the basis of arterial blood gas analysis and is, therefore, used infrequently in the field. (See ACLS algorithms in Appendix A.)

Contraindications

None in confirmed metabolic acidosis.

Precautions

Infiltration can cause tissue necrosis.

Interactions

Sodium bicarbonate can inactivate catecholamines and precipitate calcium preparations when administered in the same IV line.

Dosage

Adults: 1.0 mEq/kg given initially as an IV bolus; half the initial dose may be repeated every 10 minutes.
Children: The initial dose is the same as the adult dose. Thereafter it should be administered on the basis of arterial blood gas analysis.[7]

Administration

Sodium bicarbonate is administered by IV bolus. In adults and children a 8.4% solution (1 mEq/ml) is used. In neonates a 4.2% solution (0.5 mEq/ml) should be used.

◆ Verapamil (Calan, Isoptin)

Verapamil is a calcium channel blocker.

Mechanism of action

Calcium channel blockers inhibit the influx of calcium across the cell membrane of cardiac and vascular smooth muscle cells. The ultimate effect of this action is:

- decreased AV conduction
- decreased sinoatrial automaticity
- dilated coronary and systemic arteries
- decreased cardiac contractility

Indications

Verapamil is indicated in the treatment of narrow complex PSVTs that do not require cardioversion. It is also indicated in atrial fibrillation and atrial flutter to control rapid ventricular response.

Contraindications

- hypotension
- sinus bradycardia
- AV block

Precautions

Because verapamil reduces the force of contraction, it should be used with great caution in patients with CHF. Use of verapamil should be avoided in patients with Wolff-Parkinson-White (WPW) syndrome. If used for patients with WPW syndrome who have PSVT, the patient should be monitored very closely and a defibrillator should be available. It should be used with caution in patients with history of hepatic or renal insufficiency (dosage reduction is recommended).

Side effects

- bradycardia
- hypotension
- AV block
- headache
- may induce or exacerbate CHF

Interactions

Verapamil interacts with many other drugs. When given concurrently with digoxin, serum digoxin levels are increased, placing the patient at risk for digitalis toxicity. Verapamil should not be given concurrently with IV beta-adrenergic blocking agents because additive effects can result in hypotension, bradycardias, and dysrhythmias.

Dosage

For treatment of dysrhythmias, verapamil is administered in the following dosages:

Adults: 2.5 to 5 mg given as IV bolus over 2 minutes; doses can be repeated at 5 to 10 mg every 15 to 30 minutes up to a total of 20 mg.

Children: verapamil should not be used in infants because cardiovascular collapse has been reported in association with its use.[3] Its use is also discouraged in children because it can cause hypotension and myocardial depression.[7]

Elderly: dose should be the lower range of normal (2 to 4 mg) over a slower period of time (3 to 4 minutes).[6]

Administration

For treatment of supraventricular tachydysrhythmias, verapamil should be injected undiluted into a patent IV of D_5W, Ringer's lactate, or normal saline. Continuous ECG and blood pressure monitoring must be done during and after IV administration of verapamil. Emergency drugs to counteract serious side effects (bradycardia and hypotension) should be immediately available. Atropine, beta-adrenergics, and IV calcium are effective in the treatment of overdosage or severe side effects. Because of the additional effect of vasodilation, postural hypotension is a frequent sequelae to IV dosage. Patient should be kept recumbent for at least 1 hour after IV dosage.

9

Neurologic Emergencies

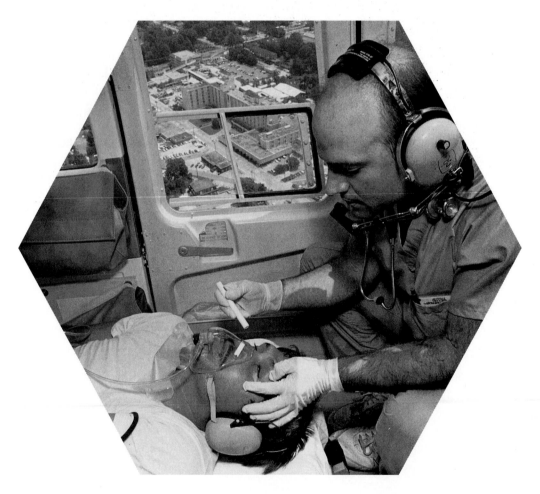

OBJECTIVES

1. Describe the role of oxygen administration in the management of neurologic trauma.
2. Explain the use of mannitol in patients with head injuries.
3. Describe the use of methylprednisolone in patients with spinal cord injuries.
4. Explain the circumstances under which drugs are administered for the treatment of seizures.
5. List three drugs used in the prehospital management of seizures.
6. Describe the pharmacologic management of comas of unknown origin.

Neurologic emergencies are those emergencies that involve some alteration in the function of the nervous system. Signs and symptoms vary widely according to the specific etiology but generally involve changes in level of consciousness or motor function. Neurologic emergencies can present even the most experienced paramedic with difficulties in early recognition and management.

For the purposes of this chapter neurologic emergencies are categorized as either traumatic or nontraumatic. Traumatic emergencies include injury to the brain or spinal cord. The discussion of nontraumatic emergencies is limited to the pharmacologic management of seizures. This chapter also discusses the pharmacologic management of comas of unknown origin.

◆ CASE PRESENTATIONS

Case Presentation 1 (Seizure)

Paramedics are dispatched at 9 PM to a residence for a "child having seizures." The dispatcher attempts to calm the 14-year-old baby-sitter who placed the call. The dispatcher reports the following information to the paramedics while they are en route to the child's home. The patient is a 3-year-old female with "full body shaking." There is no known past medical history, and no medications have been taken. The baby-sitter states that the child feels feverish and her skin appears "gray." The baby-sitter reports that she cannot feel any respirations while the child is seizing.

The paramedics enter the home 7 minutes after the initial call carrying oxygen and a medic box. The patient appears to be in the clonic phase

DRUGS PROFILED IN THIS CHAPTER		
CLASSIFICATION	DRUG	PAGE
Anticonvulsant	Diazepam	212
	Phenobarbital	215
	Phenytoin	216
Osmotic diuretic	Mannitol	213

of a tonic clonic seizure. The crew chief begins the patient assessment, while the second paramedic begins to set up the oxygen and a bag-valve mask.

The senior paramedic asks the baby-sitter if the child has been seizing the entire time since she placed the call to 9-1-1. The baby-sitter replies that the child stopped for a while and then began again. The sitter also reports that the child has been healthy, has never before had a seizure, and is not taking any medication. The sitter has notified the child's parents.

The paramedics ventilate the child with 100% oxygen via bag-valve mask and contact medical direction for orders. The medical direction physician orders an IV of Ringer's lactate at a keep-open rate and diazepam in slow, 0.5-mg incremental boluses to a maximum of 2.5 mg.

Case Presentation 2 (Coma of Unknown Origin)

Paramedics are dispatched at 7:30 PM to a home where an unknown medical emergency exists. The paramedic crew arrives in 8 minutes to find the front door open and a woman calling for them to come up to the second floor. They notice that the house is clean and odorless.

The patient is a 60-year-old man who is lying in bed and is unresponsive to verbal and painful stimuli. There are no outward signs of trauma. The patient is incontinent. His vital signs are: P-142 (thready), R-28 (full and regular), and BP-140/78. He appears to weigh approximately 190 lb. His breath has no distinct odor. The patient is flaccid in all extremities. His pupils are dilated to 8 mm bilaterally and unresponsive to light.

One paramedic administers oxygen via face mask at a rate of 10 L/min and asks the patient's wife if the patient has experienced anything similar to this in the past. His wife replies that he has not. The history provided by the wife indicates that the patient has been unconscious since she placed the call to 9-1-1. He has no history of recent illness or surgery, has not had an accident, and has not complained of feeling badly.

The paramedics insert an oropharyngeal airway, monitor the patient's cardiac rhythm (sinus tachycardia), and prepare to start an IV of D_5W. After cannulating the left antecubital vein, a blood drop is placed on a dextrose reagent strip to obtain a blood sugar level. The IV is then run at a keep-open rate. The dextrose strip indicates that the blood sugar level is approximately 70 mg/dl.

After contacting medical direction, the paramedics intubate the patient and assist ventilations with 100% oxygen. They secure the patient onto a long spine board, making sure to include the extremities. They then administer an IV bolus of 50 ml of $D_{50}W$ with no response. They follow the $D_{50}W$ with 100 mg of thiamine IV. After the thiamine is administered, they administer naloxone at 1-mg boluses every 3 minutes up to a total of 10 mg. ◆

PHARMACOLOGIC MANAGEMENT OF TRAUMATIC NEUROLOGIC EMERGENCIES

Traumatic injuries that affect the brain and/or spinal tissue require effective, immediate supportive care. Such measures include spinal stabilization, airway protection, oxygen administration, ventilatory assistance, and circulatory support. Because much of the damage that occurs with head and spinal injuries occurs secondarily as a result of inflammation and edema, attention should also be given to the prevention or reduction of cerebral and spinal edema.

Head Injury

Management of patients with head injuries focuses on maintaining adequate tissue oxygenation and cerebral blood flow and reducing or preventing increases in cerebral edema, thereby decreasing intracranial pressure.

The pharmacologic agent most frequently used in the prehospital management of traumatic head injuries is oxygen. (Refer to Chapter 7 for a discussion of oxygen administration.) Hyperventilation with 100% oxygen provides a simple, fast, and effective means of reducing cerebral edema.

Oxygen administration serves a two-fold purpose as both **hypoxia** and **hypercarbia** tend to worsen cerebral edema. First, increased oxygenation of hypoxic brain tissue results in cerebral vasoconstriction and, subsequently, decreased intracranial pressure. Second, hyperventilation with an adequate rate (24 to 30 breaths per minute) and volume (800 ml) reduces carbon dioxide tension, further reducing cerebral edema.[14] However, hyperventilation at too rapid a rate can decrease carbon dioxide blood levels to the extent that excessive cerebral vasoconstriction occurs and cerebral perfusion is reduced to harmful levels.

Mannitol (Cystosol, Cytal), a potent osmotic diuretic, is also used to reduce cerebral edema in patients with head injuries. Mannitol works by drawing fluids from the interstitial and intracellular spaces into the vasculature, thereby reducing cerebral edema and decreasing intracranial pressure. It is, however, used *infrequently* in the prehospital setting and only after aggressive airway management with 100% oxygen and positive-pressure ventilation has been initiated and a thorough physical assessment has ruled out any life-threatening conditions other than head injury.

Mannitol should be administered cautiously in the prehospital setting for several reasons. First, it can cause a more rapid expansion of intracranial hematomas. Second, individuals with head trauma usually have a high potential for other life-threatening traumatic injuries, and the signs and symptoms associated with these other injuries are often concealed. Unlike other diuretics, mannitol produces diuresis even when renal circulation is reduced, such as during hypovolemic shock, trauma, or dehydration. Thus its use in patients with head trauma complicated by hypovolemia is contraindicated.[1] Finally, because mannitol causes an increase in intravascular volume, the potential for rapid onset of respiratory distress exists for patients with preexisting congestive heart failure or traumatic chest injuries.

In the past, dexamethasone, a synthetic steroid, was given in the prehospital setting to patients with head injuries to prevent cerebral edema. Dexamethasone is no longer used in head trauma cases because its action is poorly understood. Additionally, dexamethasone has sodium retention properties that result in water retention.

Spinal Injury

The prehospital management of patients with spinal cord injuries has not traditionally included the administration of drugs other than oxygen and IV fluids. More recently, the administration of methylprednisolone, a glucocorticoid, has shown promise in significantly improving neurophysiologic capability.[6] Although methylprednisolone is not yet routinely used in the prehospital setting, clinical trials have been conducted and its use may become more prevalent in the future.

Most of the tissue damage and subsequent paralysis in spinal cord injury is a result of localized inflammation. This inflammation causes mechanical damage, loss of electrical activity through nerve cell membranes, and loss of adequate blood flow and oxygen supply. Methylprednisolone reduces inflammation and suppresses immune responses through numerous actions. As a result of its smaller molecular size, methylprednisolone passes through cell membranes more quickly, resulting in higher serum concentrations when compared with other glucocorticoids.[6,11]

Studies have shown that a 30 mg/kg IV bolus of methylprednisolone should be administered over 15 minutes (2 g in a 70-kg patient) within 8 hours following a spinal cord injury.[6] This bolus should be followed by an IV infusion of 5.4 mg/kg/hr over 24 hours (a total of 8 more grams for a typical patient). No significant reversal of neural deficit has been noted in patients who received initial drug therapy after 8 hours.[6] The therapeutic benefits of methylprednisolone are not seen immediately following spinal injury (most initial doses are given 6 to 8 hours following injury) but instead are evident months later.[6]

PHARMACOLOGIC MANAGEMENT OF NONTRAUMATIC NEUROLOGIC EMERGENCIES

Many types of nontraumatic neurologic emergencies are seen in the prehospital setting. Examples include cerebrovascular accidents (CVAs), transient ischemic attacks (TIAs), drug overdoses, poisonings, electrolyte imbalances, metabolic disturbances, and seizures. Prehospital management of these emergencies is directed primarily at supporting adequate ventilation and circulation. With the exception of seizures, pharmacologic intervention is usually limited to the administration of oxygen and IV fluids.

Seizure medications are administered in the field only when major motor seizures are persistent and potentially life-threatening or in cases of **status epilepticus.** Drugs should not be administered in the prehospital setting for a single, isolated seizure. For example, the patient in Case Presentation 1 clearly required pharmacologic intervention. The seizure was persistent and the change in skin color and lack of chest rise indicated respiratory compromise.

Pediatric seizures can be caused by fever, hypoxia, infection, head trauma, hypoglycemia, electrolyte imbalances, poisonings, congenital deformities, tumors, or epilepsy. Case Presentation 1 presented evidence of a febrile seizure. The case illustrates that, regardless of the specific etiology, initial management remains the same: protect the patient from injury, provide adequate ventilation and oxygenation, and obtain IV access. If there is evidence of recurrent seizure activity with life-threatening complications or if status epilepticus exists, drug administration is indicated.

Diazepam (Valium) is the drug of choice for the prehospital management of status epilepticus or other persistent, recurrent seizures. Diazepam belongs to a group of drugs called **benzodiazepines**.

Diazepam is the benzodiazepine used most frequently in the prehospital setting. Diazepam has several pharmacologic actions, including muscle relaxation, antianxiety, sedative, hypnotic, and anticonvulsant properties.

Diazepam is used in the prehospital setting for its antianxiety and anticonvulsant effects. Because diazepam is a controlled substance and is frequently abused by health-care professionals and patients, paramedics are responsible for appropriate documentation of the drug's use.

Although most advanced life support services carry diazepam as the first-line anticonvulsant, an alternative benzodiazepine that is sometimes used in the field is lorazepam (Ativan). Studies suggest that lorazepam maintains an effective therapeutic plasma concentration for several hours without noticeable delay in onset of action.[9] Diazepam, on the other hand, is rapidly distributed to the brain, providing a plasma concentration that declines rapidly with an initial half-life of 10 to 15 minutes. However, diazepam still remains the drug of choice in convulsive emergencies because it is effective in controlling up to 90 percent of these episodes, regardless of seizure type or cause.[9]

Phenytoin (Dilantin) and phenobarbital (Luminal) are anticonvulsants that are used far less frequently than diazepam in the prehospital setting. Both may be used to suppress recurring seizure activity after the administration of diazepam. Prehospital health-care providers should keep in mind that many patients chronically take oral preparations of phenytoin or phenobarbital for prevention of seizure activity. Thus IV loading doses of either drug can potentially result in toxic serum drug levels. To prevent this possible complication a careful history of the present illness and past medical history should be obtained to preclude any potential problems.

Another important consideration is that these anticonvulsants are incompatible with many other drugs. In addition, each of them is likely to precipitate when combined with water solutions such as D_5W. For these reasons anticonvulsants should ideally be injected directly into the vein. However, this is rarely done in actual practice. An alternative method is to flush the IV tubing with normal saline before and after administration of anticonvulsants. Additionally, the injection site on the administration tubing should be as close to the insertion site as possible.

PHARMACOLOGIC MANAGEMENT OF COMAS OF UNKNOWN ORIGIN

Comas of unknown origin present a significant challenge to paramedics. Because coma can result from numerous conditions (see box) and depress the reflexes that protect the airway, a sound primary survey, aggressive airway management, and early oxygen delivery should be top priorities. As soon as possible, paramedics should search for the cause of the coma, using information gathered in a secondary survey, a check of environmental surroundings, and an interview with family members or bystanders. Before contacting medical direction for consideration of parenteral drug intervention, the paramedics in the Case Presentation 2 used this approach in an attempt to find a cause of their patient's coma.

COMMON CAUSES OF COMA

Structural:

Trauma
Brain tumor
Epilepsy
Intracranial hemorrhage

Metabolic:

Anoxia
Hypoglycemia
Diabetic ketoacidosis
Hepatic failure
Renal failure
Thiamine deficiency

Respiratory:

Chronic obstructive pulmonary disease
Inhalation of toxic gas

Cardiovascular:

Hypertensive encephalopathy
Shock
Anaphylaxis
Dysrhythmias
Cardiac arrest
Cerebrovascular accident

Drugs:

Barbiturates
Narcotics
Hallucinogens
Depressants (including alcohol)

Infections:

Meningitis
Encephalitis

From Bledsoe BE, Porter RS, Shade BR: *Paramedic Emergency Care*, Englewood Cliffs, NJ, 1991, Prentice Hall.

KEY TERM

Coma—a state of deep unconsciousness in which the patient cannot be awakened and is not responsive to verbal and painful stimuli.

After providing supportive care and oxygen administration, the traditional management of patients with comas of unknown origin includes the administration of $D_{50}W$, thiamine, and naloxone.[1,3,5,7,12] Hypoglycemia is a serious medical emergency. (Refer to Chapter 10 for a complete discussion on the management of hypoglycemia.) If the cause of coma is unknown and the serum glucose level cannot be determined, $D_{50}W$ should be administered.

Thiamine (vitamin B_1) should be administered prior to or just after the administration of $D_{50}W$ in patients with comas of unknown origin. Thiamine prevents the occurrence of severe neurologic symptoms in patients who are given $D_{50}W$ in the presence of thiamine deficiency. Thiamine deficiency can result from alcoholism and malnutrition. This deficiency can rob the body of significant amounts of energy extracted from glucose because thiamine is required for production and utilization of glucose. Severe thiamine deficiency can reduce glucose utilization by half.[1,5]

Naloxone is typically given to patients with comas of unknown origin for potential narcotic overdose. Starting doses of 0.4 to 2.0 mg IV should be given with repeated doses administered every 2 to 3 minutes. If the patient does not respond (as evidenced by improved respiratory function) after administration of 10 mg, it is unlikely that the coma is caused by narcotic overdose.[12]

In Case Presentation 2 the cause of the patient's condition was unclear. The actions of the paramedics in this case illustrate the prehospital management priorities: protecting the airway, improving tissue oxygenation, supporting circulation, and protecting cervical spine alignment unless trauma can definitely be ruled out. The patient in this case was placed on a long spine board and secured (including extremities) before drug administration, because patients often display violent reactions when aroused from a coma.

SUMMARY

The initial management of traumatic head or spinal cord injuries includes airway maintenance, ventilation, oxygenation, spinal immobilization, and support of circulation. Oxygen administration has proven effective in reducing intracranial pressure through a decrease in cerebral edema. Although mannitol is also effective in reducing cerebral edema, it is given infrequently in the prehospital setting because of its potential side effects. The early administration of high-dose steroids, such as methylprednisolone, has been effective in decreasing neural deficits in spinal trauma and may be used in prehospital medicine in the future.

IV diazepam is the drug of choice for initial control of persistent seizure activity in the prehospital setting. Phenytoin and phenobarbital have also proven to be useful for patients with recurring seizures.

In cases of comas of unknown origin, oxygen, $D_{50}W$, thiamine, and naloxone can usually be administered safely in the field.

The most vital and important function of prehospital personnel faced with neurologic emergencies is fast and efficient supportive care. Proper airway management techniques and oxygen administration cannot be overemphasized during prehospital care as central nervous system tissue is quickly damaged with oxygen deprivation. Only after supportive care does cautious, parenteral drug administration become truly effective.

REFERENCES

1. Abrams AC: *Clinical drug therapy—rationales for nursing practice*, ed 3, Philadelphia, 1991, JB Lippincott.
2. Alfaro-Lefevre F et al: *Drug handbook—a nursing approach*, Redwood City, Calif, 1992, The Benjamin/Cummings Publishing Co.
3. Allen A, editor: *Advanced emergency care for paramedic practice*, Philadelphia, 1992, JB Lippincott.
4. Bledsoe BE, Bosker G, Papa FJ: *Prehospital emergency pharmacology*, ed 3, Englewood Cliffs, NJ, 1992, Prentice Hall.
5. Bledsoe BE, Porter RS, Shade BR: *Paramedic emergency care*, Englewood Cliffs, NJ, 1991, Prentice Hall.
6. Bracken MB et al: A randomized control trial of methylprednisolone or naloxone in the treatment of acute spinal-cord injury, *N Engl J Med* 322:1405, 1990.
7. Caroline NL: *Emergency care in the streets*, ed 3, Boston, 1987, Little, Brown & Co.
8. Deglin JH, Valerand AH, Rssin MM: *Davis's drug guide for nurses*, ed 2, Philadelphia, 1991, F.A. Davis.
9. Gilman AG, editor: *The pharmacological basis of therapeutics*, ed 8, New York, 1990, Pergamon Press.
10. Greenwald J: *The paramedic manual*, Englewood, Colo, 1988, Morton Publishing Co.
11. Halpern JS: Administering methylprednisolone for acute spinal cord injuries, *J Emerg Nurs* 17:1, 1991.
12. Levy DB: Update on naloxone—use in the prehospital setting, *J Emerg Med Serv* 12(12):36, 1987.
13. Mathewson MK: *Pharmacotherapeutics*, Philadelphia, 1986, F.A. Davis.
14. McSwain NE, editor: *Pre-hospital trauma life support*, ed 2, Akron, Ohio, 1990, Educational Direction.
15. Peppers MP: Spinal cord injury and methylprednisolone, *Emerg* 24:6, 1992.
16. Skidmore-Roth L: *Mosby's nursing drug reference*, St Louis, 1991, Mosby–Year Book.

The authors wish to acknowledge Richard K. Walker for his contribution to this chapter.

DRUG PROFILES
◆ Diazepam (Valium)

Diazepam belongs to a group of drugs called benzodiazepines, which are nonbarbiturate sedative-hypnotic drugs (minor tranquilizers). Diazepam is a potent anticonvulsant used for acute cases of persistent tonic-clonic seizures or status epilepticus.

Mechanism of action

Therapeutic effects of diazepam include cessation of seizure activity, relief of anxiety, skeletal muscle relaxation, and induction of amnesia.

Diazepam's exact mechanism of action is uncertain; however, it probably increases the seizure threshold through potentiation of an inhibitory neurotransmitter (gamma-aminobuteric acid), which decreases neural cell activity in all regions of the central nervous system. Anxiety is decreased by inhibiting cortical and limbic arousal. Diazepam promotes muscle relaxation through inhibition of spinal motor reflex pathway.

Indications

- Short-term control of severe convulsive seizures
- Status epilepticus
- Premedication prior to cardioversion
- Acute anxiety states
- Skeletal muscle relaxant
- Management of symptoms of alcohol withdrawal

Contraindications

- Patients in various states of shock, coma, or respiratory depression
- Patients who have used other central nervous system depressants, including alcohol

Precautions

Diazepam should be given cautiously to patients with hepatic dysfunction, renal insufficiency, or any history of drug addiction. With the elderly or debilitated patient, a dose reduction is usually required.

Side effects

Side effects of diazepam include central nervous system and cardiovascular manifestations ranging from a simple headache to cardiac arrest. Frequent major side effects include respiratory depression, apnea, and hypotension. For this reason, resuscitative equipment should be readily available. Frequent minor side effects include dizziness, ataxia, fatigue, confusion, and transient drowsiness.

Interactions

Diazepam should not be mixed with any other drugs or IV solutions. If direct IV injection is not feasible, the drug should be administered through an infusion tubing as close to the insertion site as possible. In addition, the infusion tubing should be flushed with normal saline before and after administration.

Dosage

Onset of action of diazepam is 1 to 5 minutes, with peak actions between 5 to 10 minutes and duration of effects lasting from 15 to 60 minutes.

Adults: Seizure activity—5 to 10 mg IV (may be repeated every 15 to 30 minutes, up to a total of 30 mg). An alternative method is to give the drug in 2-mg increments until seizure activity is controlled.
Anxiety—2 to 5 mg IV
Cardioversion—5 to 15 mg IV

Infants and Children: Seizure activity—1 month to 5 years: 0.2 to 0.5 mg slow IV push every 2 to 5 minutes to a maximum of 5 mg;
5 years and older: 1 mg slow IV push every 2 to 5 minutes to a maximum of 10 mg

Administration

Diazepam should be administered by slow IV push not to exceed 5 mg per minute in adults. In children the total dose should be administered over a 2 to 5 minute period. Its onset of action and peak effects follow minutes after administration with duration of action from 15 to 60 minutes. In the absence of IV access, diazepam can be administered intraosseously or rectally.

As with the administration of any central nervous system depressant, the patient's respirations, pulse, and blood pressure should be monitored frequently throughout therapy. The large veins of the forearm are preferred as injection sites to the small veins of the dorsal aspect of the hand because of the local venous irritation that occurs with IV administration.

◆ Mannitol (Cystosol, Cytal)

Mannitol is primarily used in the prehospital setting to decrease intracranial pressure from cerebral edema by promoting systemic diuresis. This compound is a naturally occurring, six-carbon sugar that exhibits osmotic diuretic properties.

Mechanism of action

With its large molecular size, mannitol remains in the intravascular space drawing water from the cerebral tissues into the bloodstream, thereby decreasing intracranial pressure.

Indications

- Acute cerebral edema

Contraindications

- Severe pulmonary congestion/pulmonary edema
- Congestive heart failure
- Hypovolemia
- Active intracranial bleeding

Precautions

Caution should be used when administering mannitol to patients with limited cardiac reserve, elderly patients, and patients with impaired renal function. Safe use in pregnancy has not been established.

Side effects

The most common side effect of mannitol is hypovolemia from excessive diuresis. Other side effects are related to inadequate urinary output and fluid overload. Rapid administration can precipitate transient volume expansion, resulting in congestive heart failure.

Interactions

Mannitol is incompatible with most other drugs. It is compatible with D_5W, Ringers lactate, and normal saline.

Dosage

Adults: 1.5 to 2.0 g/kg of a 15% to 25% solution IV over 30 to 60 minutes
Children: 1 to 2 g/kg of 15% to 20% solution IV over 30 to 60 minutes.
Begin with low dose and increase based on patient's condition.

Administration

Mannitol is normally administered by IV infusion or slow IV bolus. The onset of diuresis following IV administration is 20 to 60 minutes. Peak effects are obtained from 60 to 90 minutes. An in-line filter should be used for administration because of the possibility of crystal formation in the solution. Crystallization normally begins at 45° F. If crystallization does occur, the solution may be agitated and rewarmed to dissolve crystals. Administration temperature should be as close to body temperature as possible. The infusion site should be frequently observed for infiltration because **extravasation** can lead to tissue necrosis. Finally, if an indwelling catheter is in place during long patient transports, the patient should be monitored for inadequate urinary output as well as for signs and symptoms of pulmonary overload.

◆ Methylprednisolone (See page 156)

◆ Naloxone (See page 272)

◆ Phenobarbital

Phenobarbital is a barbiturate that is used in prehospital medicine as an anticonvulsant. Like phenytoin, it has a relatively slow onset of action (15 to 30 minutes) and is used for seizures that are refractory to diazepam or as a maintenance drug after diazepam administration.

Mechanism of action

Phenobarbital produces central nervous system depression, including sensory cortex depression, decreased motor activity, and alteration of cerebellar function. Its exact mechanism of action is unclear; however, its effects may result from interference with transmission of impulses at the cerebral cortex along with depression of the reticular activating system. As with phenytoin, phenobarbital increases seizure threshold at the cerebral cortex level.

Indications

Phenobarbital has many therapeutic uses. The indications specifically related to prehospital administration include:
- Treatment of major motor seizures and complex partial seizures
- Recurrent or complicated febrile seizures in children
- Status epilepticus

Contraindications

- Pregnancy
- Severe respiratory depression

Precautions

Because of phenobarbital's effect on the central nervous system, the drug should be given cautiously to patients who have respiratory or cardiac deficiencies. Caution should also be taken with patients with renal impairment, hepatic dysfunction, and diabetes mellitus. In elderly patients dosage reduction is usually necessary. Safe use has not been established during pregnancy or for nursing mothers.

Side effects

Phenobarbital's side effects include drowsiness, dizziness, headache, residual sedation (hangover), respiratory depression, hypotension, and paradoxical excitement in children and the elderly.

Interactions

Phenobarbital should not be administered through an IV tubing with any other drugs. An additive effect should be expected when given with other central nervous system depressants, such as alcohol, antihistamines, narcotics, and other sedative/hypnotics.

Dosage

Adults: 10 to 20 mg/kg not to exceed a rate of 60 mg/min. In severe cases it may be given up to a total of 20 mg/kg.

Children: 15 to 20 mg/kg not to exceed a rate of 60 mg/min. In severe cases it may be given every 10 to 15 minutes up to a maximum of 20 mg/kg.

Administration

In the prehospital setting phenobarbital should be administered via slow IV push or by IV infusion. It can be diluted with D₅W, Ringer's lactate, or normal saline. For IV administration, onset of action is approximately 5 minutes, with peak effects occurring in approximately 30 minutes. Large veins should be used for administration because of the alkalinity of the solution.

During administration, the patient's respiratory and cardiovascular status should be frequently monitored. Because of the risk of cardiovascular collapse and apnea, resuscitation equipment should be easily accessible.

◆ Phenytoin (Dilantin)

Phenytoin has a much slower onset of action than diazepam and is normally used after diazepam administration for recurring seizure activity. It has also been used to maintain seizure suppression after diazepam administration because diazepam is short-acting.

Mechanism of action

Phenytoin limits the spread of seizure activity in the motor cortex, possibly through a decrease in neurosynaptic transmission. It also increases seizure threshold at the cerebral cortex level. As an antidysrhythmic, it decreases excitability, automaticity, and conduction velocity of the myocardium. Phenytoin actually increases conduction through the atrioventricular node by increasing the atrioventricular node refractory period.

Indications

- Treatment and prevention of tonic clonic seizures and complex partial seizures
- Status epilepticus
- Control of dysrhythmias, particularly those related to digitalis toxicity

Contraindications

- Sinus bradycardia
- All degrees of heart block

Precautions

Because of phenytoin's effects on the myocardium, it should be used cautiously in patients with hypotension, myocardial insufficiency, or heart failure. Cautious use should also be maintained in patients with impaired liver or kidney function, alcoholism, diabetes mellitus, hyperglycemia, and respiratory depression. Safe use in pregnancy has not been established.

Side effects

- Respiratory depression
- Central nervous system manifestations, with drowsiness, blurred or double vision, slurred speech, headache, and confusion being most frequent
- Hypotension with rapid IV administration

Interactions

Phenytoin should not be administered with D_5W because of the possibility of precipitation. Caution should also be exercised when used in conjunction with other drugs as many drugs can increase or decrease phenytoin serum levels.

Dosage

Adults: 700 to 1000 mg IV (15 to 18 mg/kg) not to exceed a rate of 50 mg/min, for status epilepticus.
Children: 15 to 20 mg/kg IV not to exceed a rate of 1 to 3 mg/kg/min.

Administration

In emergency settings phenytoin is always given via the IV route. Due to its incompatibilities with many drugs and most IV solutions, it should be given only in normal saline. During administration, the largest vein possible should be used because of the possibility of tissue irritation from the alkalinity of the solution. For IV administration, onset of action is from 2 to 30 minutes, with peak effects occurring in 1 to 3 hours. The patient should be monitored closely for signs of toxicity because a narrow margin exists between the therapeutic and toxic serum levels. As with other anticonvulsants, resuscitation equipment should be available because of the potential of respiratory depression, apnea, or cardiac arrest.

primarily by regulating the transport of glucose across the cell membrane where it is used for energy. When insulin is not available, glucose is not transported into the cells in sufficient quantities, and the serum glucose level rises.

Diabetes mellitus is classified into two types: Type I and Type II. Table 10-1 compares these types of diabetes mellitus. Type I, **insulin-dependent diabetes mellitus (IDDM)**, formerly referred to as juvenile-onset diabetes, is characterized by the absence of insulin production and an acute onset of symptoms. While IDDM occurs most often in patients under the age of 30, it can occur in patients of any age. Patients with IDDM are dependent on the administration of insulin injections for survival.

Type II, **noninsulin-dependent diabetes mellitus (NIDDM)**, formerly referred to as adult-onset diabetes, is characterized by a slow onset and usually occurs in adults over the age of 40. With NIDDM there is impaired production of insulin by the pancreas and/or a decrease in the cellular response to insulin.

Patients with NIDDM are managed by diet, exercise, and oral hypoglycemic agents. Oral hypoglycemic agents stimulate the production of

Table 10-1 Features of Insulin-Dependent Diabetes Mellitus (IDDM) and Noninsulin-Dependent Diabetes Mellitus (NIDDM)

	IDDM	NIDDM
Synonym	Type I	Type II
Age of onset	Usually < 30	Usually > 40
Onset of symptoms	Sudden (symptomatic)	Gradual (usually asymptomatic)
Body weight	Usually nonobese	Obese (80%)
Incidence	10%	90%
Insulin-dependent	Yes	Usually not required
Insulin-resistant	No	Yes
Receptors	Normal	Usually decreased or defective
Plasma insulin	Decreased	Normal or increased
Complications	Frequent	Frequent
Ketoacidosis	Prone to	Usually resistant
Diet	Mandatory	Mandatory

From McKenry LM, Salerno E: *Mosby's pharmacology in nursing*, St Louis, 1992, Mosby–Year Book.

insulin in the pancreas and work only in patients who have some pancreatic function. Oral hypoglycemic agents are not artificial forms of insulin.

If diet, exercise, and oral hypoglycemic agents fail to maintain normal levels of serum glucose, patients with NIDDM may be required to take insulin at various times. Some noninsulin-dependent patients eventually progress to become insulin-dependent.

The primary goal of treatment in patients with both types of diabetes mellitus is to balance the intake of insulin or other hypoglycemic agents with dietary intake and exercise. Failure to maintain this balance can result in acute complications. Inadequate or excessive food intake, excessive exercise, incorrect doses of insulin, or physiologic stresses, such as infection or illness, can cause dramatic fluctuations in serum glucose levels. Abnormally high serum glucose (hyperglycemia) or abnormally low serum glucose (hypoglycemia) levels can present life-threatening emergencies.

HYPOGLYCEMIC EMERGENCIES

Hypoglycemia is a clinical syndrome that occurs when the serum glucose level falls below the normal range. It is often characterized by a sudden onset and rapid progression. Patients usually become symptomatic at serum levels below 45 mg/dl (2.5 mOsm/L). However, signs and symptoms can be related to how rapidly the blood sugar falls, rather than to an absolute numerical value. *Because glucose is necessary for normal cellular function, particularly in the brain, hypoglycemia is a serious emergency that must be assessed and managed quickly.* **Failure to do so can result in severe neurological impairment and even death.**

Although hypoglycemia can occur with both Type I and Type II diabetes mellitus, it occurs more commonly in patients who take insulin. It is, in fact, often referred to as an insulin reaction. There are a number of insulin products available today with variations in onset, peak, and duration of action.[9] A knowledge of the various types of insulin (Table 10-2) is useful when assessing the diabetic patient. Determining the time and type of the patient's last insulin injection will help in differentiating hypoglycemia from hyperglycemia, as hypoglycemic reactions are more likely to occur during peak periods of insulin activity.

Factors that can precipitate hypoglycemia in patients who take insulin are excessive exercise, decreased dietary intake, alcohol consumption, incorrect dosage of insulin, or a change in the site of injection. Hypoglycemia can be precipitated in noninsulin-dependent patients when there are imbalances in dietary intake and oral hypoglycemic agents. Hypoglycemia rarely occurs in nondiabetic patients.

Table 10-2 Characteristics of Insulin Preparations

INSULINS*	ONSET (HOURS)	PEAK EFFECT (HOURS)	DURATION OF ACTION (HOURS)
Rapid Acting			
Insulin injection (Regular Insulin) †	½-1	2-4	5-7
Prompt insulin zinc suspension (Semilente)	1	2-6	12-16
Intermediate Acting			
Insulin zinc suspension (Lente Insulin)	1-3	8-12	18-28
Isophane insulin suspension (NPH Insulin)	3-4	6-12	18-28
Isophane insulin suspension (70%) plus insulin injection (30%) (Mixtard, Novolin 70/30)	½	4-8	24
Long-Acting			
Extended insulin zinc suspension (Ultralente)	4-6	18-24	36
Protamine zinc insulin suspension (PZI)	4-6	14-24	36

From McKenry LM, Salerno E: *Mosby's pharmacology in nursing*, St Louis, 1992, Mosby–Year Book.
*All above insulins, with the exception of Mixtard, Novolin combinations, are available in 40-unit and 100-unit strengths. Beef, pork, beef-pork, and human insulins are available in rapid-acting insulins and the three insulins listed under Intermediate Acting. The others are animal sources only.
†This is the only insulin for intravenous use. Intravenously, the onset of action is within ⅙ to ½ hour, and duration of action within ½ to 1 hour.

The signs and symptoms of hypoglycemia are caused by altered cerebral function (the brain depends on glucose for energy and normal metabolism) and activation of the autonomic nervous system.[6] Early changes in mental status may be subtle, such as restlessness or inability to concentrate. As glucose levels fall, slurred speech, irritability, and even combative or bizarre behavior can develop. Hypoglycemia is easily mistaken for drug or alcohol intoxication or psychosis. As hypoglycemia progresses, the patient may experience seizures or coma. Activation of the autonomic nervous system results in hunger, nausea, anxiety, sweating, tachycardia, and peripheral vasoconstriction.

Signs and symptoms of hypoglycemia vary widely among individuals but generally follow the same pattern in one individual. Table 10-3 compares the signs and symptoms of hypoglycemia and hyperglycemia.

The pharmacologic management of hypoglycemia consists of the administration of oxygen, initiation of an IV of D$_5$W at a keep-open rate, and administration of an agent to raise serum glucose levels. These agents include oral forms of glucose, 50% dextrose solution (D$_{50}$W), and glucagon. Ideally, a baseline blood sample should be drawn and hypoglycemia confirmed by use of a glucose **reagent** strip or **capillary blood glucose measuring device** *prior* to the administration of any of these agents. In situations in which glucose reagent strips or capillary blood glucose measuring devices

Table 10-3   Signs and Symptoms of Hypoglycemia and Hyperglycemia

SIGNS AND SYMPTOMS	HYPOGLYCEMIA	HYPERGLYCEMIA	
		DIABETIC KETOACIDOSIS	HYPEROSMOLAR NONKETOTIC SYNDROME
Onset	Acute, occurs over several minutes	Gradual, occurs over several hours or days	Gradual, occurs over several hours or days
Neurologic	Headaches, dizziness, confusion, difficulty concentrating, bizarre behavior; seizures and coma in severe cases	Restlessness, headache, coma (seen less often than with hyperosmolar nonketotic syndrome)	Stuporous, comatose, seizures
Respiratory	Normal or shallow respiration	Kussmaul's respirations; acetone (fruity) odor on breath	No odor on breath
Cardiovascular			
Pulse	Normal or rapid	Weak, rapid	Weak, rapid
Blood pressure	Normal	Normal or low	Low
Gastrointestinal	Hunger, drooling	Anorexic, nausea and vomiting, excessive thirst	Weight loss, nausea and vomiting, excessive thirst, excessive hunger
Genitourinary	Not remarkable	Increased urination leading to dehydration	Increased urination leading to dehydration
Skin	Pale, cool, clammy	Dry, warm	Dry, warm

are not available and hypoglycemia is suspected, a blood specimen should be drawn for analysis in the emergency department, and the appropriate form of glucose should be administered on the basis of the patient's history and presenting signs and symptoms.

If the patient is conscious, cooperative, and has a gag reflex, glucose can be administered orally. This can be in the form of food or liquids that contain glucose, such as candy, carbonated beverages, and sweetened orange juice, or using commercially available glucose paste.

If the patient's level of consciousness is altered to the extent that administering an oral form of glucose would compromise airway patency, glucose should be given intravenously in the form of $D_{50}W$. For example, in Case Presentation 1, the IV route was clearly indicated by the patient's altered level of consciousness (e.g., failure to respond to verbal commands).

Fifty milliliters of $D_{50}W$ contains 25 g of dextrose. IV administration of dextrose is the most rapid and definitive treatment for hypoglycemia.

The patient's response to a bolus of $D_{50}W$ is usually immediate and dramatic. However, the actual rise in the serum glucose level from one 50 ml bolus of $D_{50}W$ varies. In one study, the change in glucose levels among 51 patients ranged from a low of 37 mg/dl to a high of 370 mg/dl.[1] **Researchers point out that, when only one 50 ml bolus of $D_{50}W$ is given, there is the potential for continued hypoglycemia.**[1] Patients should be monitored closely for signs and symptoms of continued hypoglycemia and the bolus repeated if necessary.

Hypoglycemic patients who receive $D_{50}W$ may awaken and refuse further care. Prehospital providers must inform these patients of the need for further evaluation and treatment in the hospital, as done in Case Presentation 1. If the patient adamantly refuses further care and transport, careful documentation and compliance with local guidelines for communication with medical direction must be followed.

When the patient's condition precludes the oral administration of glucose and IV access cannot be obtained, intramuscular administration of glucagon provides an alternative to giving glucose.[5] Glucagon is a hormone that raises the serum glucose level by stimulating the breakdown of glycogen, a stored form of glucose, in the liver. To be effective, adequate glycogen stores must be present. Glucagon is not effective in the treatment of prolonged or profound hypoglycemia in which glycogen stores have been depleted.

Hypoglycemia is a serious emergency that requires rapid intervention to avoid permanent neurologic deficits. Hypoglycemia should be considered as a possible causative factor in any situation in which there is an unexplained change in the patient's level of consciousness.

HYPERGLYCEMIC EMERGENCIES

Hyperglycemia exists when there is a greater than normal amount of serum glucose in the blood. The condition occurs most often in patients with diabetes mellitus but can also occur in neonates and with the administration of steroids. In diabetic patients, hyperglycemia may lead to diabetic ketoacidosis (DKA) or hyperosmolar nonketotic syndrome (HNKS). The primary pathology in both conditions is profound dehydration resulting from the osmotic diuresis caused by hyperglycemia.

Diabetic Ketoacidosis

DKA can be caused by inadequate insulin intake, physical or emotional stress, or undiagnosed diabetes. The patient in Case Presentation 2 had suffered a recent physical illness and had reduced her dosage of insulin. As with this case, DKA is most likely to occur in Type I diabetes; however, it is occasionally seen in Type II diabetes during severe illness or stress.

In the absence of insulin, glucose cannot be used for cellular energy. The resulting cellular starvation causes the breakdown of fats and protein for use as energy sources. As fats are degraded, free fatty acids (FFAs) are released. When FFAs are metabolized in the liver, **ketones** are formed. The accumulation of ketones causes acidosis that is manifested by a decrease in pH. Proteins are the last source of energy to be used. The process of converting protein to a cellular energy source (gluconeogenesis) results in dramatically increased serum glucose and nitrogen levels. Eventually, the extremely high glucose levels lead to profound osmotic diuresis and electrolyte loss. Vomiting is frequently caused by the acidosis, adding to the fluid volume deficit. The patient's skin becomes dry and the eyes appear sunken. Hypotension, accompanied by a rapid, thready pulse, is also a result of profound dehydration.

As illustrated in Case Presentation 2, the management of DKA in the prehospital setting focuses on providing oxygen, supporting the vital signs, and treating dehydration. Patients may require as much as 6 to 10 liters of IV fluids to replace fluid loss. The fluid of choice is normal saline at a rate of 200 to 500 ml/hour. Hypotonic saline (0.45 percent) can also be used.

Insulin is not administered in the field as a function of routine emergency care. Insulin is, however, an important component of treatment in the hospital setting.

Hyperosmolar Nonketotic Syndrome

HNKS occurs in Type II diabetics who are able to produce enough insulin to prevent the fat and protein degradation that occurs with DKA. Insulin levels are not sufficient to prevent severe hyperglycemia and osmotic diuresis. Symptoms of HNKS are usually **insidious**. Because these patients do not have the gastrointestinal upset associated with ketosis, they are not alerted to seek medical attention. They may tolerate **polydipsia** and **polyuria**

KEY TERMS

Ketones—normal metabolic products (β-hydroxybutyric acid and aminoacetic acid); excessive production of these occurs in uncontrolled diabetes mellitus.

Polydipsia—excessive thirst.

Polyuria—excessive urinary output.

for weeks, with hyperglycemia and dehydration worsening with delayed treatment. Eventually, neurological symptoms (e.g., altered mental status, seizures, hemiparesis, and coma) usually alert family and friends to the need for medical attention. Because of these typical delays in treatment, hyperglycemia and dehydration associated with HNKS are usually more severe than that seen with DKA. HNKS is a life-threatening emergency, with mortality rates ranging from 5 to 30 percent.[8]

Although there are characteristic differences between HNKS and DKA (Table 10-3), these may be difficult to discern in the field.[2] However, the prehospital management of HNKS is the same as that for DKA.

DIFFERENTIATING HYPOGLYCEMIA FROM HYPERGLYCEMIA

When it is not possible to obtain a patient's blood glucose level, particularly if the patient is unresponsive, paramedics should administer $D_{50}W$. The administration of 25 g of dextrose (50 ml of $D_{50}W$) will not adversely affect the patient in DKA or HNKS. In contrast, failure to treat severe hypoglycemia can result in neurologic damage or even death.

In the unconscious patient, where etiology is unknown and history does not specifically point to either hypoglycemia or hyperglycemia, the patient should be given $D_{50}W$. When the unconscious patient does not respond to $D_{50}W$, other causes must be considered. See Chapter 9 for a complete discussion of Coma of Unknown Origin.

SUMMARY

Diabetes mellitus is a common cause of medical emergencies. The majority of medical emergencies related to diabetes mellitus involve hypoglycemia. Other diabetic emergency conditions are associated with hyperglycemia, which can cause DKA or HNKS.

Hypoglycemia is treated with the administration of oral glucose or intravenous $D_{50}W$. The administration of $D_{50}W$ to patients with severe hypoglycemia can be life-saving. There are few circumstances in which paramedics will see such a dramatic response to drug therapy.

Although insulin is the definitive treatment for hyperglycemic emergencies, it is generally not administered in the prehospital setting. Prehospital intervention for severe hyperglycemia is focused on treatment of the hypovolemia that results from dehydration.

Both hypoglycemic and hyperglycemic emergencies can result in altered levels of consciousness. Prehospital management of these patients consists of providing oxygen and IV fluids, and supporting vital functions. When patients exhibit altered levels of consciousness and the serum glucose level is unknown, D$_{50}$W should be administered. Dextrose will not cause harm or significantly alter the clinical status of the hyperglycemic patient, but it may prove to be life-saving for the patient with severe hypoglycemia.

REFERENCES

1. Adler PM: Serum glucose changes after administration of 50% dextrose solution: pre- and in-hospital calculations, *Amer J Emerg Med* 4(6):504, 1966.
2. Bledsoe BE: Dealing with diabetic emergencies, *J Emerg Med Serv* 16(12):40, 1991.
3. Madigan KG: *Prehospital emergency drugs pocket reference*, St Louis, 1990, Mosby–Year Book.
4. McKenry LM, Salerno E, Hamelink MC: *Mosby's pharmacology in nursing*, ed 7, St Louis, 1989, Mosby–Year Book.
5. Miller K: Dextrose, thiamine, and glucagon, *Emerg* 16, February 1987.
6. Porth CM: *Pathophysiology—concepts of altered health status*, ed 3, Philadelphia, 1990, JB Lippincott.
7. Shannon MT, Wilson BA, Stang CL: *Govoni and Hayes drugs and nursing implications*, ed 7, Norwalk, Conn, 1992, Appleton & Lange.
8. Smeltzer SC, Bare BC: *Brunner and Suddarth's textbook of medical and surgical nursing*, Philadelphia, 1992, JB Lippincott.
9. Steil C, Deakins DA: Today's insulins: what you and your patient need to know, *Nurs 90* 20(8):34, 1990.
10. Taigman M: Just a little sugar—serious talk about d-50, *J Emerg Med Serv* 33, 1988.

DRUG PROFILES
◆ 50 Percent Dextrose Solution

Dextrose, also referred to as glucose, is a **monosaccharide** metabolized by the cells of the body for energy. There are 25 g of dextrose in 50 ml of $D_{50}W$.

Mechanism of action

$D_{50}W$ increases blood glucose levels when administered intravenously.

Indications

$D_{50}W$ is indicated in hypoglycemia to restore normal blood glucose levels, and in coma or seizures when etiology is unknown.

Contraindications

Intracranial hemorrhage and cerebral vascular accident are considered contraindications for the administration of $D_{50}W$; however, it is not always possible to diagnose these conditions accurately in the field. Therefore, when a patient experiences an acute onset of altered mental status and blood glucose levels are not available, hypoglycemia should be suspected and $D_{50}W$ administered. There are no contraindications for the administration of $D_{50}W$ to patients who are unconscious and suspected of having hypoglycemia.

Precautions

The administration of $D_{50}W$ can precipitate severe neurologic impairment (Wernicke-Korsakoff's syndrome) in alcoholic patients. This syndrome is related to a thiamine deficiency that occurs with alcoholism. Thiamine should be administered to patients with a history of alcoholism prior to the administration of $D_{50}W$. Refer to page 210 for a discussion on administration of thiamine.

Side effects

Side effects of $D_{50}W$ are related to the hypertonicity and acidity of the solution and include pain, warmth, and burning upon administration. Phlebitis, sclerosis, and thrombosis of the vein can occur.

Interactions

There are no significant drug interactions.

Dosage

Adults: 25 to 50 g (50 to 100 ml of 50 percent solution)

Infants and Children: 0.5 to 1 g/kg of a 25 percent solution ($D_{25}W$); a 50 percent solution may be diluted 1:1 with normal saline or sterile water

Administration

$D_{50}W$ is administered intravenously. It is available in preloaded syringes containing 50 ml of a 50% solution of dextrose (25 gm). Because of the high glucose content and its hypertonicity, $D_{50}W$ can cause phlebitis and sclerosis of the vein in which it is administered. With infiltration, tissue necrosis can occur. It is crucial that 50 percent dextrose be given in a free-flowing IV line, preferably through a large-bore catheter in a large vein. In addition, $D_{50}W$ should be given slowly over at least 3 minutes.[10] The vein should be flushed copiously with D_5W or normal saline during and after administration. During administration, the plunger of the syringe can be drawn back to determine patency.[3]

◆ Glucagon

Glucagon is a hormone secreted by the alpha cells of the pancreas. It provides an alternative to $D_{50}W$ when IV access is not possible and alterations in the patient's level of consciousness preclude the use of oral forms of glucose.

Mechanism of action

Glucagon increases blood glucose by stimulating the breakdown of glycogen (stored form of glucose) in the liver; inhibiting the conversion of circulating glucose to glycogen; and stimulating glucose metabolism in the liver (gluconeogenesis). The action of glucagon is dependent on the liver breaking down glycogen (glycogenolysis); therefore, it is ineffective in patients with liver dysfunction or inadequate glycogen stores, as seen with chronic states of hypoglycemia or starvation.

Indications

Hypoglycemia.

Contraindications

Allergy to proteins.

Precautions

Glucagon should be administered cautiously to patients with cardiovascular disease because it has both positive **inotropic** and **chronotropic** properties. Caution should be exercised in patients with known hepatic or renal insufficiency.

Side effects

Glucagon is generally well-tolerated. Nausea and vomiting are the most common reactions to the drug and are related to dosage.

Interactions

None.

Dosage

Adults: 0.5 to 1 mg (1 mg = 1 USP unit)
Infants and Children: 0.025 mg per kg body weight up to a maximum of 1 mg
If glucagon is ineffective in waking the patient in 5 to 20 minutes, the dose may be repeated up to two additional doses.[7]

Administration

Glucagon is available in a powder that must be reconstituted prior to administration. It can be administered intravenously, intramuscularly, or subcutaneously. The onset of action with IV administration is within 1 to 2 minutes and within 5 to 20 minutes with intramuscular administration. Although glucagon can be administered intravenously, its use in the field is primarily an alternative to $D_{50}W$ when IV access is not possible. In such situations, it is usually administered intramuscularly. The subcutaneous route is not generally used for the emergency management of hypoglycemia.

◆ Glucose (Glutose, Insta-Glucose)

Glucose is a monosaccharide that is given orally and is readily absorbed in the intestine.

Mechanism of action

After absorption from the gastrointestinal tract, glucose is readily distributed in the tissues and provides a prompt increase in circulating blood sugar. The onset of action is approximately 10 minutes.

Indications

Hypoglycemia.

Contraindications

None.

Precautions

Because changes in levels of consciousness can change rapidly in patients with hypoglycemia, it is important to ascertain the patient's ability to swallow an oral preparation of glucose without airway compromise.

Side effects

Nausea.

Interactions

None.

Dosage

Adult: 10 to 20 g; may be repeated in 10 minutes if necessary
Infants and Children: only under medical direction

Administration

Glucose is available in a paste and is administered orally. **It must be swallowed because it is not absorbed sublingually or buccally.**

He quickly completes a primary survey of the mother and baby and finds the mother to be frightened, confused, pale, and diaphoretic. Vital signs are: P–weak and thready at 128/min; R–32/min and shallow; and BP–84/42 mm/Hg. Pulse oximetry shows a hemoglobin saturation of 97 percent. There is blood on the bedding, but the amount is difficult to estimate. The baby is crying actively with a pulse of 130 and a respiratory rate of 36.

One of paramedics determines that the baby is doing well and directs his partner to dry and warm the newborn, and then clamp and cut the umbilical cord. The first paramedic then completes his assessment of the mother.

The paramedic places the newborn on the mother's breast to begin suckling. He notes the mother is still pale and diaphoretic. He places her on oxygen at 6 L/min via a nasal cannula and obtains a second set of vital signs: P–136; R–32; and BP–76/40 mm Hg. An external inspection indicates that vaginal bleeding is continuing. The paramedic instructs his partner to massage the patient's fundus and to let him know if it becomes firm and if the bleeding stops. Upon consulting medical direction, the paramedic establishes an IV of 1000 ml of lactated Ringer's using a standard solution set and a 16 gauge, over-the-needle catheter.

The bleeding fails to be controlled by fundal massage and having the baby nurse. Another set of vital signs reveals: P–144; R–36; and BP–70/36 mm Hg. The patient is now responsive to painful stimuli only. Transport time to the hospital is approximately 25 to 30 minutes. Medical direction orders 20 units of oxytocin to be infused initially at a rate of 10 ml/min and thereafter titrated to uterine response and severity of bleeding. A second IV of lacated Ringer's is started for volume replacement.

En route to the hospital, the vaginal bleeding stops and the patient's level of consciousness begins to improve after 10 minutes. The rate of oxytocin administration is gradually decreased, and the patient's response is monitored. The lactated Ringer's is run wide open for the remainder of the trip to the hospital.

Case Presentation 2 (Preeclampsia)

A 25-year-old female in the seventh month of her first pregnancy calls her physician at 3:15 AM complaining of a headache and abdominal cramping. She had gained approximately 4 to 8 lb at her prenatal visit one week prior, at which time her blood pressure was 138/96 mm Hg. She has a history of high blood pressure and takes an antihypertensive agent daily. Her doctor advises her to call an ambulance and go to the emergency department where he will meet her.

County Rescue 6 arrives at the house in 7 minutes and one of the paramedics performs a rapid assessment. He notes that the patient has marked edema. Her vital signs are: P–90; R–24; and BP–170/106 mm Hg. She complains of "feeling funny and seeing flashes of light." The paramedic starts oxygen at 6 L/min via a face mask and calls medical direction for orders. Medical direction orders an IV of 5 percent dextrose in water at a keep open rate and magnesium sulfate 1 g by IV bolus to suppress any possible seizures. The patient is transported immediately, and magnesium sulfate is administered en route to the hospital. ◆

POSTPARTUM BLEEDING

Although some bleeding is expected following childbirth, excessive blood loss can lead to hypovolemia. By definition, excessive postpartum bleeding refers to blood loss of more than 500 ml. It is, however, difficult to accurately determine the exact volume of blood loss in the field. In addition to direct observation of the bleeding, paramedics should assess all postpartum patients for signs of hypovolemia: tachycardia, diminished or thready peripheral pulses, decreased level of consciousness, and rapid, shallow respirations.

In the prehospital setting, postpartum bleeding should be managed initially by administering oxygen and IV fluids (usually lactated Ringer's or normal saline), gently massaging the fundus of the uterus to increase uterine tone, and allowing the baby to nurse. As a last resort, medication may be required.

For example, the paramedic in Case Presentation 1 attempted to manage the patient's hypovolemia by having the baby nurse, having his partner massage the patient's fundus, and administering oxygen and IV fluids. Despite these interventions, the patient's blood pressure continued to drop and her level of consciousness deteriorated. At this point, it was appropriate for the paramedics to consider drug administration.

The drug of choice for uncontrolled, excessive **postpartum bleeding** is oxytocin (Pitocin, Syntocinon). Due to the potentially serious side effects seen with oxytocin, such as cardiac dysrhythmias and uterine rupture, it is preferable that it be administered in a hospital setting. However, persistent and excessive bleeding that does not respond to other measures may necessitate its use in the field.[6] Medical direction and/or local protocols should be consulted prior to administering oxytocin.

Oxytocin should be administered **only after the baby and placenta have been delivered and the possibility of multiple births has been ruled out.** Oxytocin should be administered with great caution and judicious monitoring of the patient's response. If possible, oxytocin should be administered via an infusion pump or other accurate control device. If these are not readily available in the field, a minidrip and volume control chamber should be used, with the IV flow rate monitored very closely.

TOXEMIA OF PREGNANCY

Toxemia of pregnancy is an abnormal condition of unknown etiology. Often referred to as pregnancy-induced hypertension, it can have serious manifestations, such as preeclampsia and eclampsia. Preeclampsia is a form of toxemia characterized by hypertension, edema, headaches, and visual disturbances. Eclampsia, the gravest form of toxemia, is characterized by major motor seizures and/or coma.

The prehospital management of patients with suspected preeclampsia includes providing a quiet and dimly lit environment to prevent seizure activity and establishing an IV of D_5W at a keep-open rate. Magnesium sulfate is used to control seizures associated with severe preeclampsia and eclampsia.

The major concern for the patient in Case Presentation 2 was the high risk for an imminent seizure. The history of hypertension coupled with a first pregnancy, edema, recent weight gain, and abdominal pain were consistent with preeclampsia. The complaint of a visual aura (seeing flashes of light) signaled the imminent possibility of seizure. The administration of magnesium sulfate decreased the likelihood of a seizure in this patient.

Because the adverse reactions of magnesium sulfate, such as respiratory depression and complete heart block, are serious, paramedics must be prepared to manage them. The necessary airway management equipment and calcium gluconate, which can be used to reverse the effects of magnesium sulfate, should be readily available.

Diazepam can also be used to control seizures in patients with preeclampsia and eclampsia. Refer to page 212 for a drug profile for diazepam.

NEONATAL RESUSCITATION

When deliveries occur in the prehospital setting, paramedics must be prepared to care for the neonate as well as the mother. Resuscitation of neonates is aimed at the restoration of normal cardiopulmonary function. The American Heart Association uses an inverted pyramid (Figure 11-1) to illustrate the frequency of interventions required in neonatal resuscitation. A majority (about 80 percent) of neonates require only positioning, suctioning of the airway, maintenance of temperature, and tactile stimulation.[2] Those

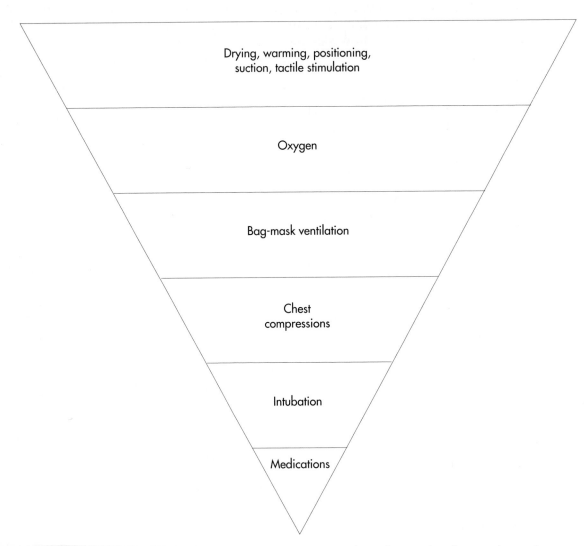

Drying, warming, positioning, suction, tactile stimulation

Oxygen

Bag-mask ventilation

Chest compressions

Intubation

Medications

Figure 11-1   Inverted pyramid reflecting the approximate relative frequencies of neonatal resuscitative efforts. Note that a majority of infants respond to simple measures. Most infants requiring chest compression will usually require intubation, and these efforts are often performed simultaneously. (From American Heart Association: *Textbook of advanced cardiac life support*, ed. 2, Dallas, 1990, American Heart Association.)

who do require further intervention usually respond to oxygen administration and bag-valve mask ventilation. Only a very small percentage of neonates require drug therapy.[2]

Drugs are indicated in neonatal resuscitation when adequate ventilation with 100 percent oxygen and chest compressions for 30 seconds fail to establish a heart rate of at least 80 beats per minute. Medications that may be required during neonatal resuscitation include epinephrine, sodium bicarbonate, dopamine, and naloxone hydrochloride.

Epinephrine is indicated in asystole or for a heart rate less than 80 that has not responded to adequate ventilation with 100 percent oxygen and chest compressions. Sodium bicarbonate is administered for the treatment of acidosis only in cases of prolonged arrest that don't respond to other resuscitative measures or when profound metabolic acidosis is confirmed by laboratory analysis. Refer to page 199 for a drug profile for sodium bicarbonate.

Dopamine is used infrequently, but may be required to support blood pressure. Refer to page 187 for a drug profile for dopamine. Naloxone hydrochloride is administered for respiratory depression associated with narcotic use by the mother. Refer to page 272 for a drug profile for naloxone hydrochloride. Table 11-1 outlines neonatal dosages and routes of administration.[2]

Table 11-1 Drugs Used in Neonatal Resuscitation

DRUG	INDICATION	DOSE
Dopamine	Hypotension	5 µg/kg/min initially by IV infusion; may increase to 20 µg/kg/min if necessary
Epinephrine	Asystole or heart rate less than 80 after adequate ventilation with 100% oxygen	0.01-0.03 mg/kg IV (0.1-0.3 ml of a 1:1000 solution); repeated every 3 to 5 minutes
Naloxone	Respiratory depression associated with the mother receiving narcotics within 4 hours of delivery	0.1 mg/kg; may repeat every 2 to 3 minutes
Sodium bicarbonate	Only in prolonged arrests that do not respond to other therapy	1 mEq/kg IV
Volume expanders (normal saline or lactated Ringer's)	Hypovolemia	10 ml/kg over 5 to 10 minutes

SUMMARY

Obstetric and neonatal emergencies rarely require pharmacologic intervention in the field. Supportive care for obstetric patients is usually sufficient to handle such emergencies. Providing oxygen, fluid, and a calm environment often go a long way toward improving patient status. Oxytocin and magnesium sulfate are only used after other methods of treatment have failed.

Neonatal resuscitation rarely requires the administration of drugs. Most neonates respond to stimulation and oxygen administration. Only when an adequate heart rate and adequate perfusion are not attainable by conservative methods are drugs administered.

REFERENCES

1. Barnhart ER: *Physician's desk reference*, ed 45, Oradell, NJ, 1991, Medical Economics Company.
2. Chameides L: *Pediatric advanced life support*, Dallas, 1990, American Heart Association.
3. Dickinson ET: Magnesium comes of age, *J Emerg Med Serv* 17(4), 1992.
4. Gahart BL: *Intravenous medications*, ed 7, St. Louis, 1991, Mosby–Year Book.
5. Gilman AG: *Goodman and Gilman's the pharmacological basis of therapeutics*, ed 8, New York, 1990, Pergamon Press.
6. Levy DB, Peppers MP, Miller K: A last resort for postpartum hemorrhage, *Emerg* 22(5):16-17, 1990.
7. Thomas CL: *Taber's cyclopedic medical dictionary*, ed 16, Philadelphia, 1989, FA Davis.

DRUG PROFILES
◆ Diazepam

See page 212.

◆ Dopamine

See page 187.

◆ Epinephrine

See page 189.

◆ Magnesium Sulfate

Magnesium sulfate is a central nervous system depressant and an anti-convulsant. As such, it has many uses. This profile emphasizes the use of magnesium sulfate in the prehospital management of severe preeclampsia and eclampsia.

Mechanism of action

Magnesium sulfate depresses the central nervous system and relaxes smooth muscle, skeletal muscle, and cardiac muscle.

Indications

- In the prehospital setting, for convulsive states associated with severe preeclampsia and eclampsia.

Contraindications

- Heart block
- Myocardial damage

Precautions

Because magnesium sulfate can cause many serious adverse reactions, calcium gluconate should be available.

Side effects

Side effects are those associated with magnesium intoxication, the most serious of which are respiratory depression and respiratory failure. Other side effects include:

- Cardiac arrest
- Circulatory collapse
- Complete heart block

- Flaccid paralysis
- Absence of knee jerk

Interactions

Magnesium sulfate is incompatible with numerous drugs. Those that have relevance in the prehospital setting are alcohol, salicylates, and sodium bicarbonate.

Dosage

The standard dose is usually 1 g of a 10 percent solution. (The dosage range is 1 to 4 g.) The smallest effective dose should be used.

Administration

In preeclampsia or eclampsia, magnesium sulfate should be administered by slow IV push only.

◆ Naloxone Hydrochloride

See page 272.

◆ Oxytocin (Pitocin, Syntocinon)

Oxytocin is a hormone secreted by the posterior pituitary gland in response to the suckling action of a baby at the mother's breast. Although oxytocin occurs naturally, a synthetic preparation is available for use.

Mechanism of action

Oxytocin causes rhythmic contraction of uterine smooth muscle. Contraction of uterine smooth muscle decreases bleeding from uterine vessels.

Indications

- In the prehospital setting, for excessive postpartum bleeding only.
- In the hospital setting, to induce labor.

Contraindications

Although there are a number of contraindications to the use of oxytocin for the induction of labor, there are none in the management of excessive postpartum bleeding.

Precautions

In the prehospital setting, oxytocin should be administered only after the baby and placenta have been delivered and the possibility of multiple births has been ruled out.

Side effects

- Fluid retention (water intoxication)
- Cardiac dysrhythmias
- Anaphylaxis
- Pelvic hematoma
- Uterine spasm
- Uterine rupture
- Nausea and vomiting

Dosage

Ten to forty units in 1000 ml of D$_5$W, Ringer's lactate, or normal saline administered at a rate to control **uterine atony**. The initial rate should be 1 to 2 ml/min (60 to 120 ml/hr) titrated to the patient's response. The intramuscular dose is 3 to 10 units.

Administration

For excessive postpartum bleeding, oxytocin should be administered by IV infusion. The minimal effective dose (rate) should be used and the patient monitored for uterine response (e.g., strength, frequency, and duration of contractions and resting uterine tone). In the absence of IV access, oxytocin can be administered intramuscularly.

◆ Sodium Bicarbonate

See page 199.

12
Behavioral Emergencies

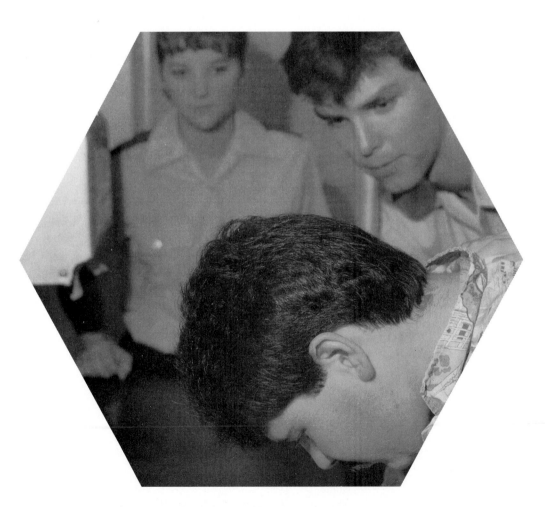

OBJECTIVES

1. List common behavioral emergencies encountered in the field.
2. Describe nonpharmacologic interventions for behavioral emergencies.
3. Discuss the use of antipsychotic agents in the prehospital setting.
4. Explain the use of diazepam in the prehospital setting.

The number of behavioral emergencies encountered by prehospital personnel has increased during the past two decades. Factors that have contributed to this increase include the trend away from the institutionalization of the mentally ill, shorter hospital stays, and increased societal stressors. Most behavioral emergencies are managed without the administration of drugs prior to the patient's arrival at the hospital. However, if the patient's behavior poses a threat to himself or to others, pharmacologic intervention by prehospital personnel may be necessary.

◆ CASE PRESENTATION

MEDIC 9 is called by a neighbor to the home of a 52-year-old male who was released from the state psychiatric hospital 6 months earlier. MEDIC 9 has transported this patient to the hospital on four previous occasions, and each time he has been violent and required antipsychotic drug intervention in the hospital emergency department. The paramedics coordinate their arrival at the scene to correspond with that of the police via radio contact.

The patient is in the house screaming and throwing objects when the paramedics arrive. The police enter the house, but the paramedics wait

DRUGS PROFILED IN THIS CHAPTER		
CLASSIFICATION	DRUG	PAGE
Antipsychotic	Haloperidol	251
Tranquilizer	Hydroxyzine	252

for them to signal safety before entering. Inside, they find the patient standing in a corner of an upstairs bedroom with his arms folded in a defiant pose. His face is taut and red with anger.

"Hi, John, I've taken you to the hospital a few times in the past month or two" begins one of the paramedics. "Would you care to go with us again?"

The patient yells obscenities at the paramedics and police, saying he isn't going anywhere and he'll stop anyone who tries to make him go. The police agree that he needs to be restrained and transported to the emergency department and will "3-0-2" him (an involuntary commitment invoked when a person is harmful to himself or others). The police officer says, "Do what you need to do. Let's get him to the hospital."

One of the paramedics contacts medical direction and gives his report. Medical direction orders the paramedics to proceed with caution, provide the minimum amount of restraint necessary to ensure patient safety, and then administer 5 mg of haloperidol intramuscularly. ◆

SPECIFIC BEHAVIORAL PROBLEMS

A behavioral emergency is one in which the patient's behavior is altered to the extent that immediate attention is required. There are a number of specific psychiatric disorders that result in altered behavior. Common examples are an acute schizophrenic episode, psychotic depression, delirium, dementia, and acute situational reaction. These disorders manifest themselves in a variety of ways: agitation, panic, fear, suicidal or homicidal thinking, and aggressive, combative, or violent behavior.

Many behavioral emergencies have physical causes, such as hypoxia, hypoglycemia, substance abuse, meningitis, or head injury. Every effort should be made to rule out a physical cause for altered behavior and to intervene appropriately.

Most behavioral emergencies can be managed and the patient transported safely without the use of medication. Initially, paramedics should employ crisis intervention and communication skills to calm the patient. If these fail to gain the patient's cooperation, the proper application of restraints to control aggressive behavior or uncontrollable patient movement may be necessary. When interpersonal methods of management and attempts at physical restraint fail to adequately control the patient's behavior, medications may be necessary.

PHARMACOLOGIC MANAGEMENT OF BEHAVIORAL EMERGENCIES

In the prehospital setting, pharmacologic intervention should be restricted to the severely agitated, combative, or acutely psychotic patient who poses a threat to himself or others and cannot otherwise be safely transported. Patients with severe behavioral disorders present a significant risk of violence and escape, and few ambulance crews have a sufficient number of people to manage a patient who is out of control.

The use of drugs to control behavior is referred to as chemical restraint. Pharmacologic treatment will vary, but it is generally intended to provide sedation. The patient in the case presentation did not respond to the paramedic's attempts to communicate with him and threatened the safety of the paramedics and the police if they attempted to physically restrain him. This is an example of a patient in need of chemical restraint.

The drug of choice for sedation of a violent or acutely psychotic patient is haloperidol (Haldol).[6,7] Haloperidol was an appropriate drug for the patient in the case presentation based on his history of psychosis and his aggressive, combative behavior. Haloperidol is a potent antipsychotic that quickly reduces tension, anxiety, and hyperactivity.[6] Haloperidol can be given orally, intramuscularly, and intravenously.[6] In the prehospital setting, haloperidol is currently being given intramuscularly. Recent studies have shown the IV route to be safe and effective in hospital settings.[6] Its IV use in the field may become more common in the future.

The **benzodiazepines** are the treatment of choice in the management of acute anxiety, panic states, and agitation associated with withdrawal from alcohol and other sedative/hypnotic drugs. Diazepam is the benzodiazepine used most frequently in prehospital medicine for behavioral emergencies because of its ability to decrease anxiety and produce sedation and hypnosis. Refer to page 212 for the drug profile of diazepam. Hydroxyzine (Vistaril) is a minor tranquilizer. It is used in cases of moderate anxiety for its sedative and antianxiety properties.

SUMMARY

Because behavioral emergencies are occurring with increasing frequency in the prehospital setting, paramedics need to be ready to manage such cases. Management may simply involve establishing rapport with the patient, or it may necessitate aggressive therapy, including physical and chemical restraint.

Sedation should be a last resort because many patients can be calmed using crisis intervention techniques and appropriate physical restraint. Should the situation call for pharmacologic intervention, drugs can help bring the patient to a more manageable state and ensure the safety of the patient and crew.

REFERENCES

1. Barnhart ER: *Physician's desk reference*, ed 45, Oradell, NJ, 1991, Medical Economics Company.
2. Factor RM: Managing the violent patient in the emergency department, *Emerg Care Q: Behav Emerg* 7(1):82-93, 1991.
3. Gahart BL: *Intravenous medications*, ed 7, St. Louis, 1991, Mosby–Year Book, Inc.
4. McKinney HE: Ethanol emergencies, *Emerg* 23(5):22-26, 1991.
5. Rice MM, Moore GP: Management of the violent patient, therapeutic and legal considerations, *Emerg Med Clin N Amer* 9(1):13-30, 1991.
6. Tutt J: New Jersey takes on Tango and Cash, *Emerg* 23(5):33-51, 1991.
7. Weiles SJ: The delirious/psychotic patient, *Emerg Care Q: Behav Emerg* 7(1):62-73, 1991.

DRUG PROFILES

◆ Diazepam

See page 212.

◆ Haloperidol (Haldol)

Haloperidol is a high-potency, fast-acting, antipsychotic agent.

Mechanism of action

Haloperidol is believed to block the stimulation of dopamine receptors.

Indications

Acute psychotic episodes.

Contraindications

- Severe toxic central nervous system depression
- Comatose state from any cause
- Parkinson's disease

Precautions

- Severe cardiovascular disorders
- Patients receiving anticonvulsant medication
- Patients receiving anticoagulants
- Patients with known allergies or with a history of allergic reactions to drugs

Side effects

Orthostatic hypotension is the most common and serious short-term side effect with parenteral administration of haloperidol.

Interactions

When used with antihypertensive agents or nitrates, haloperidol can produce additive hypotension. Phenobarbital can decrease its effectiveness.

Dosage

For acute psychosis, 2 to 5 mg is administered intramuscularly. The dose may be repeated at 1-hour intervals until signs and symptoms are under control. For the geriatric patients, the dosage should be reduced to 0.5 to 2 mg. Haloperidol is not recommended for pediatric patients in the prehospital setting.

Administration

In the prehospital setting, haloperidol is currently administered by the intramuscular route only.

◆ Hydroxyzine (Vistaril)

Hydroxyzine is a tranquilizer used in behavioral emergencies for its sedative and antianxiety properties.

Mechanism of action

Antagonizes the action of histamine on H_1 receptors.

13

Pain Management

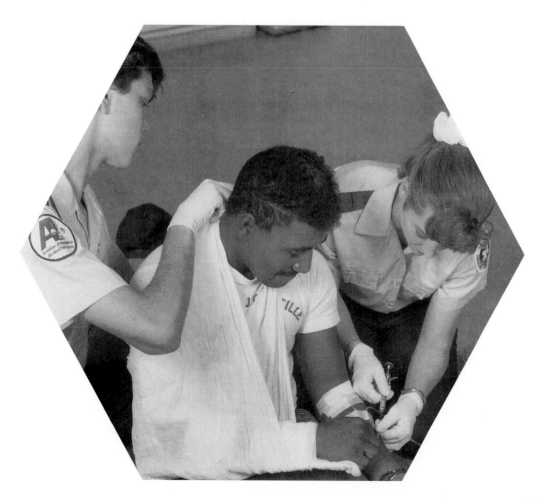

OBJECTIVES

1. Discuss the prehospital management of pain.
2. Define the term *analgesic*.
3. Explain the rationale for withholding analgesics in the prehospital setting.
4. List the drugs most commonly used for the relief of pain in the field.
5. Describe the advantages of using nitrous oxide for the relief of pain.
6. Define the term *narcotic*.
7. Differentiate between the use of morphine sulfate and meperidine in the prehospital management of pain.

The prehospital management of pain in the United States has traditionally been very conservative. In most paramedic training programs and the textbooks they use, there is little emphasis placed on providing relief of pain for patient comfort. Instead, pain is most often discussed in the context of the effects of chest pain on catecholamine levels, or as a symptom of various injuries and illnesses.

◆ CASE PRESENTATION

MEDIC 6 is dispatched to a local factory at 10:30 AM for an industrial accident involving a ruptured steam pipe that resulted in a severe burn injury.

Six minutes later, the paramedics arrive at the accident scene, where a co-worker is bent over the patient taking his pulse at the wrist. The patient appears to be about 30 years old. The co-worker looks up and

DRUGS PROFILED IN THIS CHAPTER		
CLASSIFICATION	DRUG	PAGE
Narcotic analgesic	Meperidine	259
	Morphine sulfate	260
Gaseous analgesic	Nitrous oxide	261

says, "The pipe has been secured, and the pressure's released. He got a blast of hot steam over his chest, belly, left arm, and upper left thigh. He's hurting real bad."

The patient is writhing and grimacing from the pain, and he cries out, "Help me, I can't stand it." He is pale and diaphoretic. His speech is clear and loud. The paramedics assess his chest, abdomen, and extremities, and find reddened skin and blisters forming over the burned areas. The wounds are tender and appear to be partial-thickness burns.

The paramedic crew chief does a primary and secondary survey and obtains the patient's present and past medical histories. Vital signs are: P–130 and strong; R–28 and shallow; and BP–142/80. He has not lost consciousness, vomited, or been incontinent. He reports being in good health, has had no surgeries, takes no medications, and has no known allergies.

Per local protocol, one of the paramedics prepares to administer nitrous oxide. He tells the patient, "This is oxygen and nitrous oxide. You can breathe as much of this as you want. It will help relieve the pain. If you feel nauseated or don't like the sensation, just let me know and we'll give you oxygen without the pain medication." The paramedic then contacts medical direction and receives an order for an IV of normal saline at 200 ml/hr and 10-mg morphine sulfate IV in 2-mg increments until the patient's pain is controlled.

After 8 mg of morphine sulfate is administered, the patient's pain is reduced and he is breathing easily. The transport to the hospital is uneventful. ◆

PREHOSPITAL MANAGEMENT OF PAIN

The administration of drugs to relieve pain has been somewhat limited in the prehospital setting. Traditionally, chest pain has been the only problem for which **analgesics** have been routinely given. There are a number of historically

---

KEY TERM

Analgesic—a drug that relieves pain.

sound reasons for this, the most important being the potential masking of critical signs and symptoms when analgesics are administered. The presence of pain is often an important clue that injury has occurred. Administering analgesics in the field can interfere with an adequate assessment of the patient in the emergency department, and significant injuries may not be detected in a timely fashion. Additionally, the patient's level of consciousness can be altered by analgesics, making assessment of the patient difficult.

Much of prehospital pain management is limited to providing comfort measures, such as positioning, splinting, and the use of cold packs. When these measures are not sufficient, such as in cases in which untreated pain can **exacerbate** the patient's condition before arrival at the emergency department, the administration of analgesics can be incorporated into the management process. Such cases include myocardial infarction, severe burns, pain associated with kidney stones, and some musculoskeletal injuries.

The case presentation illustrates the importance of pain relief for certain patients. The relief of pain for this patient was important for several reasons: to maintain perfusion, which can be compromised in response to pain; to maintain adequate ventilation, which can be compromised with chest wall pain; and to provide comfort and relief from the pain associated with thermal burns.

The most commonly used analgesics in the field are morphine sulfate, meperidine, and nitrous oxide. The prehospital use of other agents, such as ketamine hydrochloride and fentanyl hydrochloride, has been researched and may offer valuable alternatives in the future.[4,5]

NARCOTICS

A narcotic is a drug that acts on the central nervous system to decrease the sensation of pain. Morphine sulfate and meperidine are the narcotics used most frequently in the prehospital setting.

Morphine sulfate (Duramorph) is an opiate that is derived from naturally occurring opium. It is considered to be the analgesic of choice for severe pain in the prehospital setting. It affects both the central nervous system and the cardiovascular system. Morphine is more selective than other analgesics because it binds only to the opiate receptors in the brain. It produces a potent analgesic effect and reduces the patient's emotional response to pain. The cardiovascular advantage of morphine is a reduction in the myocardial oxygen demand due to peripheral vasodilation and a subsequent decrease in systemic vascular resistance. The patient with pulmonary edema benefits from both the hemodynamic and the calming properties of morphine.

Meperidine (Demerol) is an opioid, or synthetic narcotic, that has effects similar to those of morphine. It also acts to decrease the sensation of pain, but lacks the cardiovascular advantage of morphine. Meperidine is less potent than morphine, requiring up to 10 times the dosage as morphine given parenterally to produce the same effects.[3]

Although narcotics are effective in the relief of pain, respiratory depression can result from their administration. Airway equipment should always be readily available, and adverse reactions can be reversed with naloxone, a narcotic antagonist. (Refer to page 272 for a drug profile for naloxone.)

Narcotic analgesics are most often given for severe pain when prompt relief is desired. For this reason, they are usually given intravenously. When IV access is unobtainable, the intramuscular or subcutaneous routes can be used as an alternative. However, intramuscular injections are contraindicated in patients with myocardial ischemia and/or infarction because they cause an elevation in the enzyme CPK and may confuse the diagnosis of acute myocardial infarction.

NITROUS OXIDE

Nitrous oxide is a safe and effective analgesic gas when self-administered via a demand valve in a 50:50 mixture with oxygen. As seen in the case presentation, self-administration allows the patient to determine the desired dosage and degree of relief. In addition, the drug is eliminated from the body approximately 90 seconds after administration is discontinued, nullifying the complication of masking symptoms. Nitrous oxide is also an amnesic, which helps patients forget pain.

A special precaution for the use of nitrous oxide in the prehospital setting is the need for a well-ventilated ambulance. A scavenger system, which directly removes the patient's expiratory gases from the vehicle, is recommended. Nitrous oxide has been abused as a recreational drug, and a system of strict controls should be maintained to prevent abuse by emergency personnel.

SUMMARY

The relief of pain in the prehospital setting is an important task for paramedics. The techniques for accomplishing this goal range from providing calm reassurance to pharmacologic intervention. Since pain is a very individual perception, the techniques employed will vary from call to call.

When other measures fail to relieve pain, the administration of analgesics becomes crucial. Concerns with using analgesics in the field include the risks of complications and the masking of critical signs and symptoms.

It is the responsibility of the individual paramedic to use good judgment in the area of pain relief. A sound knowledge base of the actions of the drugs used and adequate preparation for the possibility of adverse reactions are a must for instituting pharmacologic therapy.

REFERENCES

1. Barnhart ER: *Physician's desk reference*, ed 45, Oradell, NJ, 1991, Medical Economics Company.
2. Gahart BL: *Intravenous medications*, ed 7, St. Louis, 1991, Mosby–Year Book, Inc.
3. Gilman AG: *Goodman and Gilman's the pharmacological basis of therapeutics*, ed 8, New York, 1990, Pergamon Press.
4. Myers D: Pain management the smart way, *J Emerg Med Serv* (2):46-54, June, 1992.
5. Stewart RD: Analgesia in the field, *Prehosp Disast Med* 4(1):31-34, July-September, 1989.

OBJECTIVES

1. Define the term *poison*.
2. Describe the role of poison control centers in the treatment of poisonings.
3. Discuss the use of syrup of ipecac and activated charcoal in the prehospital setting.
4. Differentiate between nonspecific and specific antidotes.
5. Explain the benefits of atropine administration in organophosphate poisoning.

Poisoning is a pathologic state resulting from the ingestion, injection, inhalation, or exposure to a poisonous substance. Potential **poisons** include elicit drugs, medications, plants, chemicals, and environmental pollutants. More than 100 million calls are made to poison control centers each year, with the majority of these calls involving children under 5 years of age.[9] Mortality from acute poisonings has been recently reported at about 12,000 deaths per year in the United States.[3] About half the deaths that occur from poisoning are intentional (suicides), whereas the other half are accidental.[3]

Poisoning can be chronic or acute. Chronic poisoning occurs when small amounts of poison are absorbed over a prolonged period of time. Acute poisoning occurs immediately, usually after a single excessive dose. Acute poisoning in children is most commonly the result of ingestion of plants, drugs, or household chemicals (usually cleaning agents). In adults, the most common cause of acute poisoning is ingestion of a central nervous system depressant, such as alcohol or a **benzodiazepine**.[3] Whether accidental or intentional, poisonings are frequently seen by paramedics. Ten percent of all emergency medical service (EMS) calls are related to poisonings.[11]

DRUGS PROFILED IN THIS CHAPTER

CLASSIFICATION	DRUG	PAGE
Adsorbent	Activated charcoal	271
Narcotic antagonist	Naloxone	272
Cholinesterase reactivator	Pralidoxime chloride	273
Emetic	Syrup of Ipecac	273

◆ CASE PRESENTATION

Unit 8 is dispatched at 8:30 AM to a commercial farm for an unconscious worker. The paramedic unit arrives to find a farm worker lying in a field near the equipment he was operating. The local fire department is already on the scene. They had been dispatched on the suspicion that the patient might have been exposed to toxic chemicals. The paramedics are provided with the appropriate protective clothing.

The paramedics assess the patient and find him to be unresponsive to verbal stimuli. They also note muscular twitching in all extremities, making it difficult to obtain vital signs. His respirations appear to be approximately 6/min and shallow. One of the paramedics begins to ventilate the patient with 100% oxygen and asks the patient's co-workers whether the patient had been using any chemicals. One of the co-workers responds that the patient had been using a pesticide. The paramedic asks the co-workers to bring the container or a material substance data safety (MSDS) form right away.

The paramedics continue ventilating the patient with 100% oxygen per bag-valve mask and place him on a cardiac monitor. The monitor shows a significant amount of artifact due to the patient's muscular twitching, but the paramedics determine the ventricular rate to be 35/min. The pulse oximeter indicates 99% hemoglobin saturation.

As they prepare an IV administration set with 500 cc of D₅W, one of the co-workers returns with a description of the contents of the pesticide used. The label indicates that the pesticide contains an organophosphate and includes emergency medical instructions to administer atropine sulfate. The fire department personnel assist in decontaminating the patient and loading him into the ambulance as quickly as possible.

After contacting medical direction, the paramedics initiate an IV and give a bolus of 1 mg atropine, followed by another 1 mg bolus 5 minutes later. While en route to the hospital, medical direction instructs the paramedics to administer 1 mg atropine every 5 minutes until the patient responds with an adequate pulse. ◆

OVERVIEW OF POISON MANAGEMENT

The first principle in the emergency response to poisonings is the same as with all emergencies: assessment of the scene for safety. Many poisonings are the result of simple ingestion and do not pose any danger to health care providers. However, any time the route of exposure to a poisonous substance is not oral, EMS personnel must recognize that exposing themselves to the substance is a potential danger and must act accordingly.

This is particularly true with substances that can be inhaled or absorbed through the skin. When the poisoning involves exposure to hazardous substances, such as a poisonous gas or liquid, paramedics must take appropriate precaution to ensure their personal safety. Although specific precautions vary according to the chemical involved, they generally include the use of protective clothing and/or a breathing apparatus. The paramedics in the case presentation would have been at significant risk of exposure had they not taken appropriate precautions, such as donning protective clothing. The fact that the patient was a farm worker who became ill suddenly with no evidence of trauma suggested the probability of toxic exposure.

The second principle in managing such an emergency is to move the patient to safety as quickly as possible while protecting the airway and cervical spine. As seen in the case presentation, the patient was moved to the ambulance at the earliest possible time.

With many poisonings, patients are not in acute distress at the time of arrival of EMS. For example, a patient who has ingested acetaminophen typically appears stable initially, and yet acetaminophen poisonings are among the most serious.

Although poisoned patients may appear stable upon arrival of EMS, life-threatening problems can quickly set in. Once unstable vital signs, respiratory distress, seizures, or impending coma are noted, stabilization and rapid transport are imperative.

Paramedics must know and follow protocols in their area for contacting and maintaining communication with the local poison control center. Most poison control centers prefer to communicate directly with the on-site providers of emergency care. This decreases any delay in treatment that could be caused by intermediate personnel relaying communication between the care provider and the poison control center. Communication with poison control involves the identification of the toxic substance, assessment of the patient, procedures for decontamination of the patient and possibly the crew, and patient management.

EMS personnel must be aware of assessment criteria that help to establish whether a poisoning has actually occurred. These include:

1. Reports of poison by the victim, family, or friends who are present. It is important for people on the scene to search for pill bottles, containers, or other information that can help establish the most likely substance responsible for the poisoning. Any containers or other evidence (i.e., substance abuse paraphernalia) should be transported along with the patient.
2. Report of history of previous poison ingestion.
3. Report of history of suicidal thoughts or expression of intent.
4. Physical characteristics, including evidence or burns around the mouth, unusual odor of the breath, discolored oral mucosa, vomitus (note appearance and odor), skin rash, diarrhea, and signs and symptoms of central nervous system excitement or depression.
5. Constant monitoring of ABCs of blood pressure.

If the victim is exhibiting signs of respiratory depression upon EMS arrival, this information must be relayed to poison control immediately. Once appropriate information has been gathered and relayed to both poison control and medical direction, treatment can be initiated. Specimens of vomitus, stool, and urine should be saved if possible and turned over to the attending physician in the emergency department for analysis.

REMOVAL AND ELIMINATION OF THE POISON

Decontamination is the removal or neutralization of a poison. Decontamination procedures have been established by the American Association of Poison Control Centers as follows[7]:

Inhaled poison—Get the victim to fresh air immediately. If the victim cannot be moved outside, all windows and doors should be opened.

Poison on the skin—Contaminated clothing should be removed. Flush the skin with water for 10 minutes, followed by gentle washing with mild soap and water.

Poison in the eye—Flush the eye with lukewarm water following the removal of contact lenses. Pour away from the unaffected eye from a container held 2 to 3 inches above the victim's eye, encouraging the victim to blink as frequently as possible during the process. Do not make any attempt to force the eyelid open. Continue this process for 15 minutes.

Swallowed poison—Call for advice. Do not administer anything by mouth prior to contacting poison control.

Household chemicals—If possible, give milk or water immediately (this is only contraindicated if the patient is unable to swallow or is having seizures). Contact poison control or medical direction.

ADMINISTRATION OF DRUGS

Nonspecific Therapy

An **antidote** is a drug or other substance that opposes the action of a poison. Only about 5% of all poison substances have specific antidotes.[3] Therefore, the drugs most often administered in the management of poisonings are considered to be nonspecific therapy. The most common of these drugs are syrup of ipecac and activated charcoal.

Syrup of ipecac is an emetic, an agent that induces vomiting. Syrup of ipecac is administered for ingested poisons. Approximately 30% of the stomach contents is emptied by vomiting following administration of ipecac.[11] Ipecac should only be given to patients who are conscious, with an intact gag reflex. It is contraindicated in cases involving the ingestion of any agent with the potential to cause a rapid onset of coma or seizures (e.g., tricyclic antidepressants) due to the risk of aspiration should the patient vomit. It is also contraindicated in cases involving the ingestion of corrosive substances, such as strong acids, alkalis (e.g., lye), or petroleum distillates (e.g., kerosene or gasoline), as vomiting can damage the esophagus. In 90% of patients, vomiting will occur within 30 minutes of ipecac administration.[3] Vomitus should be kept for analysis.

Poison control should be consulted prior to administering syrup of ipecac in the field. When possible, it is best to delay the administration of ipecac until the patient reaches the hospital. If long transport times preclude this, paramedics must take special care to be prepared to manage potential airway problems. This can be accomplished by positioning the patient appropriately and having suction equipment readily available.

Activated charcoal, an **adsorbent**, is by far the most effective agent in the nonspecific treatment of poisonings. Generally, a **slurry** of activated charcoal is administered after emesis or gastric lavage has been accomplished. Activated charcoal is becoming the drug of choice for first-line therapy in the treatment of poisonings. The trend is toward initial administration of activated charcoal due to the possible delay of activated charcoal administration if ipecac is administered first.[8] In the event ipecac is used, activated charcoal should not be administered until after vomiting has occurred, as it will adsorb the ipecac.

Specific Antidotes

A specific antidote is one that acts directly to reverse the effects of a poison. EMS providers should consult poison control and medical direction to determine whether a specific antidote should be administered. Examples of specific antidotes include benzodiazepines for tricyclic antidepressant poisonings, naloxone for opioid poisonings, and amyl nitrate for cyanide poisonings. Common situations encountered by the paramedic for which specific antidote therapy is indicated include alcohol intoxication, central nervous system depressant ingestion, and organophosphate poisoning.

Acute alcohol poisoning is usually the result of a single, excessive ingestion of ethanol over a short period of time, or ingestion of methanol, isopropyl alcohol, or ethylene glycol. These three latter substances are frequently the result of the severely debilitated alcoholic seeking less expensive alternatives to ethanol. The role of paramedics in such situations is primarily directed at identifying the substance and supporting vital functions during patient transport.

In central nervous system depressant poisonings, the patient survival may depend on the rapid identification of the substance and administration of naloxone by EMS personnel. Naloxone (Narcan) is a narcotic antagonist that works to reverse the effects of opioid central nervous system depressants. Respiratory depression and decreased levels of consciousness caused by opioids can be quickly reversed with its administration.

Organophosphate compounds are a group of chemicals used as insecticides. Due to their highly unstable chemical structure, they disintegrate within a few days and generally exhibit no cumulative effect on the environment. For this reason, they are widely used in this country as household and commercial insect sprays, in flea collars, and in agricultural applications. Because of the frequency of use of organophosphates, poisonings occur in relatively high numbers.

Organophosphates are absorbed into the body readily by all routes: dermal, respiratory, gastrointestinal, and ocular. These compounds work by inhibiting the enzyme acetylcholinesterase, which breaks down acetylcholine. When acetylcholine accumulates in the parasympathetic nervous system, all organs that it usually acts upon are overstimulated. Thus, the signs and symptoms of organophosphate poisoning include: bradycardia, hypotension, dyspnea, wheezing, blurred vision, seizure activity, and profuse sweating. A mnemonic for recognizing the signs and symptoms of organophosphate poisoning is **SLUDGE**: Salivation, Lacrimation, Urination, Defecation, Gastrointestinal distress, and Emesis. The most common cause of death due to organophosphate poisoning is respiratory arrest.

Emergency intervention for organophosphate poisoning consists of respiratory support (i.e., aggressive airway management, suctioning of secretions and administration of oxygen), antidote administration, and decontamination. Patients with organophosphate contamination should not be transported to the hospital emergency department or any closed patient area until they are decontaminated.

Once acute symptoms are under control, specific drugs may be ordered to combat the parasympathetic effects of organophosphates. One drug used for this purpose is atropine sulfate, a parasympatholytic agent that inhibits the effects of acetylcholine and reduces gastrointestinal secretions. (Refer to page 183 for a drug profile for atropine sulfate.) Another drug is pralidoxime chloride (Protopam chloride), which acts to degrade acetylcholine by reactivating the enzyme acetylcholinesterase. The result is relief of parasympathetic overstimulation. Pralidoxime chloride is used only for severe cases of organophosphate poisoning and should be administered concurrently with atropine sulfate.

SUMMARY

Poisonings occur frequently in the United States, and paramedics are often called upon to assist the victims. Treatment for these cases depends on recognition and knowledge of the type and route of poisoning.

Specific antidotes can sometimes be used when the type of poison is known. Other cases require nonspecific therapy. Whatever the case, early intervention is best.

The major concern in poisoned patients is maintenance of the airway, since respiratory depression is frequently seen. Airway equipment should be readily available to ensure proper management of this life-threatening problem.

Recognition, management, and appropriate therapy instituted at the proper time can prevent further deterioration of patient status. Poison control centers provide the best source of information for the management of acute poisonings. Paramedics should be familiar with the procedure for initiating and maintaining communication with their local poison control center.

REFERENCES

1. Barnhart ER: *Physician's desk reference*, ed 45, Oradell, NJ, 1991, Medical Economics Company.
2. Carlton FB: General management of the poisoned patient, *Emerg Care Q* 6(3):1-6, October 1990.
3. Clark JB, Queener SF, Karb VB: *Pharmacological basis of nursing practice*, ed 3, St. Louis, 1991, Mosby–Year Book.
4. DasGupta K: Antidepressant overdose, *Emerg Care Q: Behav Emerg* 7(1):29-40, April 1991.
5. Gahart BL: *Intravenous medications*, ed 7, St Louis, 1991, Mosby–Year Book.
6. Gilman AG: *Goodman and Gilman's the pharmacological basis of therapeutics*, ed 8, New York, 1990, Pergamon Press.

7. Jaser L, Crean DJ: Using the poison control center, *Emerg Care Q* 6(3):24-28, October, 1990.
8. Kirk MA, Bowers L: Cluing in on the acutely poisoned patient, *J Emerg Med Serv* 16(5):64-78, May 1991.
9. McKenry LM, Salerno E: *Mosby's pharmacology in nursing*, ed 17, St Louis, 1989, Mosby–Year Book.
10. McKinney HE: Ethanol emergencies, *Emerg* 23(5):22-26, May 1991.
11. Pruchnicki S: Just say know: recognizing the dangers of commonplace drugs, *J Emerg Med Serv* 16(2):26-42, February 1991.
12. Yealy DM et al: The safety of prehospital naloxone administration by paramedics, *Ann Emerg Med* 19(8):902-905, August 1990.

Drug Profiles

◆ Activated Charcoal

Activated charcoal is an adsorbent.

Mechanism of action

Activated charcoal adsorbs drugs and chemicals in the stomach, which prevents their adsorption into the systemic circulation. The charcoal and the adsorbed substance is then eliminated in the feces.

Indications

Poisoning by ingestion.

Contraindications

The ingestion of caustics and corrosives. It should not be used in poisonings involving strong acids, strong bases, cyanide, metals, or hydrocarbons.

Precautions

Until recently, the use of charcoal was avoided in known acetaminophen poisonings. Recent studies have shown that if the charcoal and the antidote (acetylcysteine) are given 1 to 2 hours apart adsorption of the antidote is unlikely.[10]

Side effects

Nausea and vomiting are commonly seen.

Interactions

Milk products can decrease the effectiveness of activated charcoal. Activated charcoal should not be administered before or concurrently with syrup of ipecac.

Dosage

Adults: 30 to 60 g (1 g/kg) in 8 to 16 ounces of water.
Children: 10 to 30 g (1 g/kg) in 4 to 8 ounces of water.

Administration

Orally or by nasogastric tube.

◆ Atropine Sulfate

See page 183.

◆ Naloxone (Narcan)

Naloxone is a narcotic antagonist.

Mechanism of action

Naloxone displaces narcotics from opioid receptor sites, resulting in the reversal of respiratory depression, sedation, and pupillary effects of opioid drugs. It usually works only when the central nervous system depressant ingested is an opioid.

Indications

Acutely depressed levels of consciousness. (Follow local protocol.)

Contraindications

None.

Precautions

- Pre-existing cardiac disease
- Patients who have received cardiotoxic drugs

Side effects

- Tachycardia
- Hypertension
- Hypotension
- Vomiting

Side effects are usually mild and result from the abrupt reversal of narcotic depression. Naloxone is generally viewed as very safe for administration in the field.

Interactions

None significant.

Dosage

Adults: 0.4 to 2 mg. If necessary, dose may be repeated in 2- to 3-minute intervals. If no response is observed after 10 mg, the etiology of the depressed level of consciousness should be questioned.

Neonates: 0.01 to 0.1 mg/kg (American Heart Association recommends an initial dose of 0.1 mg/kg).

Children: 1.0 mg/kg, followed by a subsequent dose of 1.0 mg/kg if no response on initial dose.

Administration

In overdoses the IV route is preferred, although subcutaneous, intramuscular, endotracheal, or intraosseous routes can be used if necessary.

◆ Pralidoxime chloride (Protopam chloride)

Pralidoxime chloride is a cholinesterase reactivator.

Mechanism of action

Pralidoxime chloride reactivates the enzyme acetylcholinesterase, which allows acetylcholine to be degraded, thus relieving the parasympathetic overstimulation caused by excess acetylcholine.

Indications

Administered concurrently with atropine sulfate in organophosphate poisonings.

Contraindications

None.

Precautions

Reduce dosage in cases of known renal insufficiency.

Side effects

- Dizziness
- Blurred vision
- Tachycardia
- Nausea
- Drowsiness
- Hyperventilation
- Muscle weakness
- Diplopia

Interactions

Pralidoxime should not be mixed in the same syringe or solution with any other drug.

Dosage

Children: 20 to 40 mg/kg.
Adults: 1 to 2 g. A second dose may be administered in 1 hour.

Administration

Given by infusion of 100 ml over 15 to 30 minutes.

◆ Syrup of Ipecac

Ipecac is an emetic.

Mechanism of action

Syrup of ipecac irritates the stomach and stimulates the vomiting center in the brain.

Indications

Poisoning in the conscious patient.

Contraindications

- Impaired level of consciousness
- Ingestion of any agent with potential to cause rapid onset of coma/seizures
- Poisonings involving acids, bases, and hydrocarbons
- Protracted vomiting

Precautions

Ipecac is cardiotoxic, but this is not a concern with the one or two doses used to induce emesis.

Side effects

Rare.

Interactions

Ipecac is adsorbed by activated charcoal. It should not be given concurrently or following the administration of activated charcoal.

Dosage

Neonates (6 months to 1 year): 7.5 to 10 ml.
Children (1 to 5 years): 15 ml.
Adults: 30 ml. The dose may be repeated once after 30 minutes if vomiting has not occurred.

Administration

Syrup of ipecac is administered orally, with up to 8 oz of water. Adult patients should be encouraged to drink 4 to 8 oz water, children 2 to 4 oz water, as this distends the stomach and makes it more susceptible to the action of ipecac. Also, if possible, have the patient walk once the ipecac is administered to help induce vomiting.

A

ACLS Algorithms

All the material contained in this appendix is reproduced with permission.

JAMA 1992; 268:2199-2275.
Copyright 1992, American Medical Association.

THE ALGORITHM APPROACH TO EMERGENCY CARDIAC CARE

These guidelines use algorithms as an educational tool. They are an illustrative method to summarize information. Providers of emergency care should view algorithms as a summary and a memory aid. They provide a way to treat a broad range of patients. Algorithms, by nature, oversimplify. The effective teacher and care provider will use them wisely, not blindly. Some patients may require care not specified in the algorithms. When clinically appropriate, flexibility is accepted and encouraged. Many interventions and actions are listed as "considerations" to help providers think. These lists should not be considered endorsements or requirements or "standard of care" in a legal sense. Algorithms do not replace clinical understanding. Although the algorithms provide a good "cookbook," the patient always requires a "thinking cook."

The following clinical recommendations apply to all treatment algorithms:

- First, treat the patient, not the monitor.
- Algorithms for cardiac arrest presume that the condition under discussion continuously persists, that the patient remains in cardiac arrest, and that CPR is always performed.
- Apply different interventions whenever appropriate indications exist.
- The flow diagrams present mostly Class I (acceptable, definitely effective) recommendations. The footnotes present Class IIa (acceptable, probably effective), Class IIb (acceptable, possibly effective), Class III (not indicated, may be harmful) recommendations.
- Adequate airway, ventilation, oxygenation, chest compressions, and defibrillation are more important than administration of medications and take precedence over initiating an intravenous line or injecting pharmacologic agents.
- Several medications (epinephrine, lidocaine, and atropine) can be administered via the endotracheal tube, but clinicians must use an endotracheal dose 2 to 2.5 times the intravenous dose.
- With a few exceptions, intravenous medications should always be administered rapidly, in bolus method.
- After each intravenous medication, give a 20- to 30-mL bolus of intravenous fluid and immediately elevate the extremity. This will enhance delivery of the drug to the central circulation, which may take 1 to 2 minutes.
- Last, treat the patient, not the monitor.

Algorithm A-1

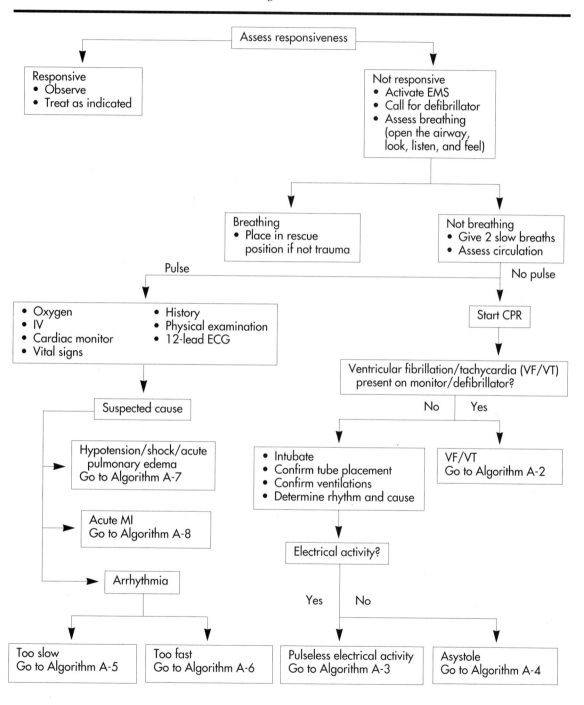

Algorithm A-1   Universal algorithm for adult emergency cardiac care (ECC).

Algorithm A-2

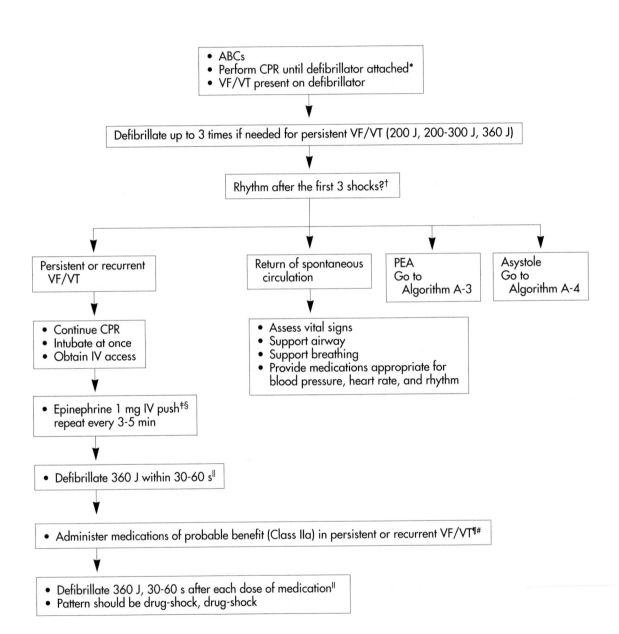

- ABCs
- Perform CPR until defibrillator attached*
- VF/VT present on defibrillator

Defibrillate up to 3 times if needed for persistent VF/VT (200 J, 200-300 J, 360 J)

Rhythm after the first 3 shocks?[†]

Persistent or recurrent VF/VT

Return of spontaneous circulation

PEA
Go to
Algorithm A-3

Asystole
Go to
Algorithm A-4

- Continue CPR
- Intubate at once
- Obtain IV access

- Assess vital signs
- Support airway
- Support breathing
- Provide medications appropriate for blood pressure, heart rate, and rhythm

- Epinephrine 1 mg IV push[†§] repeat every 3-5 min

- Defibrillate 360 J within 30-60 s[‖]

- Administer medications of probable benefit (Class IIa) in persistent or recurrent VF/VT[¶#]

- Defibrillate 360 J, 30-60 s after each dose of medication[‖]
- Pattern should be drug-shock, drug-shock

Algorithm A-2   Algorithm for ventricular fibrillation and pulseless ventricular tachycardia (VF/VT).

Class I: definitely helpful

Class IIa: acceptable, probably helpful

Class IIb: acceptable, possibly helpful

Class III: not indicated, may be harmful

*Precordial thump is a Class IIb action in witnessed arrest, no pulse, and no defibrillator immediately available.

†Hypothermic cardiac arrest is treated differently after this point. See section on hypothermia.

‡The recommended dose of **epinephrine** is 1 mg IV push every 3-5 min. If this approach fails, several Class IIb dosing regimens can be considered:

- Intermediate: **epinephrine** 2-5 mg IV push, every 3-5 min
- Escalating: **epinephrine** 1 mg-3 mg- 5 mg IV push (3 min apart)
- High: **epinephrine** 0.1 mg/kg IV push, every 3-5 min

§**Sodium Bicarbonate** (1mEq/kg) is Class I if patient has known preexisting hyperkalemia

‖Multiple sequenced shocks (200 J, 200-300 J, 360 J) are acceptable here (Class I), especially when medications are delayed

¶• **Lidocaine** 1.5 mg/kg IV push. Repeat in 3-5 min to total loading dose of 3 mg/kg; then use
- **Bretylium** 5 mg/kg IV push. Repeat in 5 min at 10 mg/kg
- **Magnesium sulfate** 1-2 g IV in torsades de pointes or suspected hypomagnesemic state or severe refractory VF
- **Procainamide** 30 mg/min in refractory VF (maximum total 17 mg/kg)

#• **Sodium bicarbonate** (1 mEq/kg IV):

Class IIa

- if known preexisting bicarbonate-responsive acidosis
- if overdose with tricyclic antidepressants
- to alkalinize the urine in drug overdoses

Class IIb

- if intubated and continued long arrest interval
- upon return of spontaneous circulation after long arrest interval

Class III

- Hypoxic lactic acidosis

Algorithm A-2—*cont'd.* (For legend see opposite page.)

Algorithm A-3

PEA includes:
- Electromechanical dissociation (EMD)
- Pseudo-EMD
- Idioventricular rhythms
- Ventricular escape rhythms
- Bradyasystolic rhythms
- Postdefibrillation idioventricular rhythms

- Continue CPR
- Intubate at once
- Obtain IV access
- Assess blood flow using Doppler ultrasound

Consider possible causes (Parentheses = possible therapies and treatments)
- Hypovolemia (volume infusion)
- Hypoxia (ventilation)
- Cardiac tamponade (pericardiocentesis)
- Tension pneumothorax (needle decompression)
- Hypothermia
- Massive pulmonary embolism (surgery, **thrombolytics**)
- Drug overdoses such as tricyclics, digitalis, β-blockers, calcium channel blockers)
- Hyperkalemia*
- Acidosis†
- Massive acute myocardial infarction (go to Algorithm A-8)

- Epinephrine 1 mg IV push,*† repeat every 3-5 min

- If absolute bradycardia (< 60 beats/min) or relative bradycardia, give **atropine** 1 mg IV
- Repeat every 3-5 min up to a total of 0.04 mg/kg§

Algorithm A-3   Algorithm for pulseless electrical activity (PEA) (electromechanical dissociation [EMD]).

Class I: definitely helpful

Class IIa: acceptable, probably helpful

Class IIb: acceptable, possibly helpful

Class III: not indicated, may be harmful

*__Sodium bicarbonate__1mEq/kg is Class I if patient has known preexisting hyperkalemia.

†__Sodium bicarbonate__ 1 mEq/kg:

Class IIa

- if known preexisting bicarbonate-responsive acidosis
- if overdose with tricyclic antidepressants
- to alkalinize the urine in drug overdoses

Class IIb

- if intubated and long arrest interval
- upon return of spontaneous circulation after long arrest interval

Class III

- hypoxic lactic acidosis

†The recommended dose of **epinephrine** is 1 mg IV push every 3-5 min. If this approach fails, several Class IIb dosing regimens can be considered.

- Intermediate: **epinephrine** 2-5 mg IV push, every 3-5 min
- Escalating: **epinephrine** 1 mg-3 mg-5 mg IV push (3 min apart)
- High: **epinephrine** 0.1 mg/kg IV push, every 3-5 min

§Shorter **atropine** dosing intervals are possibly helpful in cardiac arrest (Class IIb).

Algorithm A-3—*cont'd.* (For legend see opposite page.)

Algorithm A-4

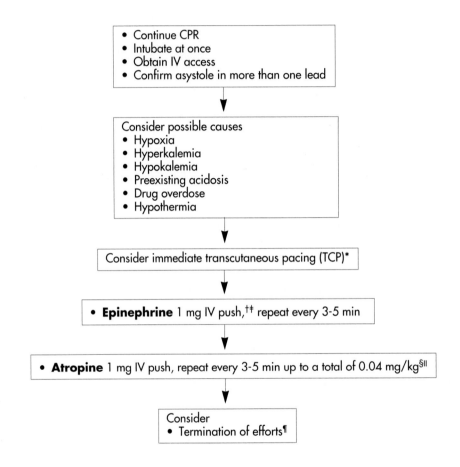

Algorithm A-4   Asystole treatment algorithm.

Algorithm A-4—*cont'd*

Class I: definitely helpful

Class IIa: acceptable, probably helpful

Class IIb: acceptable, possibly helpful

Class III: not indicated, may be harmful

* TCP is a Class IIb intervention. Lack of success may be due to delays in pacing. To be effective TCP must be performed early, simultaneously with drugs. Evidence does not support routine use of TCP for asystole.

† The recommended dose of is 1 mg IV push every 3-5 min. If this approach fails, several Class IIb dosing regimens can be considered:

- Intermediate: **epinephrine** 2-5 mg IV push, every 3-5 min
- Escalating: **epinephrine** 1 mg-3 mg-5 mg IV push (3 min apart)
- High: **epinephrine** 0.1 mg/kg IV push, every 3-5 min

‡ **Sodium bicarbonate** 1 mEq/kg is Class I if patient has known preexisting hyperkalemia.

§ Shorter **atropine** dosing intervals are Class IIb in asystolic arrest.

‖ **Sodium bicarbonate** 1 mEq/kg:

Class IIa

- if known preexisting bicarbonate-responsive acidosis
- if overdose with tricyclic antidepressants
- to alkalinize the urine in drug overdoses

Class IIb

- if intubated and continued long arrest interval
- upon return of spontaneous circulation after long arrest interval

Class III

- hypoxic lactic acidosis

¶ If patient remains in asystole or other agonal rhythms after successful intubation and initial medications and no reversible causes are identified, consider termination of resuscitative efforts by a physician. Consider interval since arrest.

Algorithm A-4—*cont'd.* (For legend see opposite page.)

Algorithm A-5

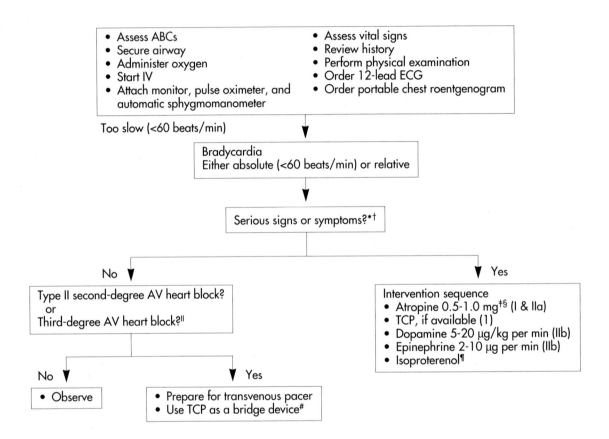

Algorithm A-5—*cont'd*

*Serious signs or symptoms must be related to the slow rate.

Clinical manifestations include:

*symptom*s (chest pain, shortness of breath, decreased level of consciousness) and

signs (low BP, shock, pulmonary congestion, CHF, acute MI).

†Do not delay TCP while awaiting IV access or for **atropine** to take effect if patient is symptomatic.

‡Denervated transplanted hearts will not respond to **atropine.** Go at once to pacing, **catecholamine** infusion, or both.

§**Atropine** should be given in repeat doses in 3-5 min up to a total of 0.04 mg/kg. Consider shorter dosing intervals in severe clinical conditions. It has been suggested that atropine should be used with caution in atrioventricular (AV) block at the His-Purkinje level (Type II AV block and new third-degree block with wide QRS complexes) (Class IIb).

‖Never treat third-degree heart block plus ventricular escape beats with **lidocaine.**

¶**Isoproterenol** should be used, if at all, with extreme caution. At low doses it is Class IIb (possibly helpful); at higher doses it is Class III (harmful).

#Verify patient tolerance and mechanical capture. Use analgesia and sedation as needed.

Algorithm A-5—*cont'd.* (For legend see opposite page.)

Algorithm A-6

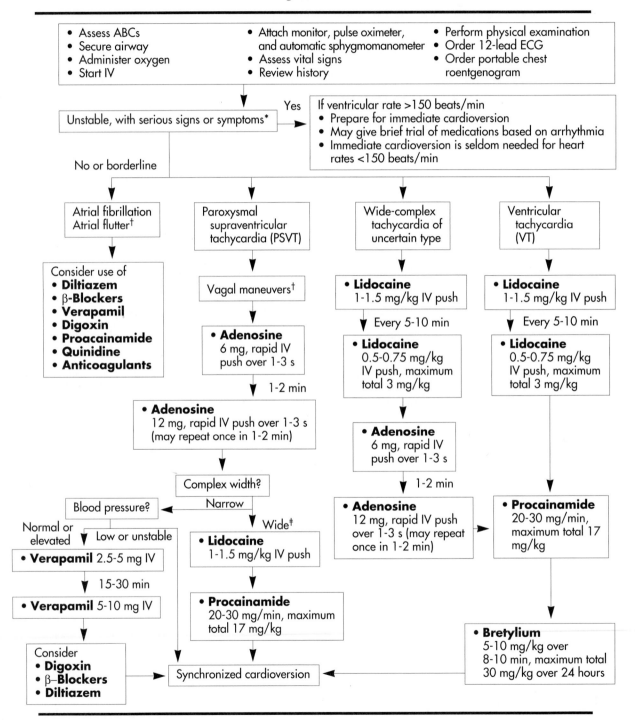

Algorithm A-6 Tachycardia algorithm.

Algorithm A-6—*cont'd*

*Unstable condition must be related to the tachycardia. Signs and symptoms may include chest pain, shortness of breath, decreased level of consciousness, low blood pressure (BP), shock, pulmonary congestion, congestive heart failure, acute myocardial infarction.

†Carotid sinus pressure is contraindicated in patients with carotid bruits; avoid ice water immersion in patients with ischemic heart disease.

‡If the wide-complex tachycardia is known with certainty to be PSVT and BP is normal/elevated, sequence can include **verapamil.**

Algorithm A-6—*cont'd.* (For legend see opposite page.)

Algorithm A-7

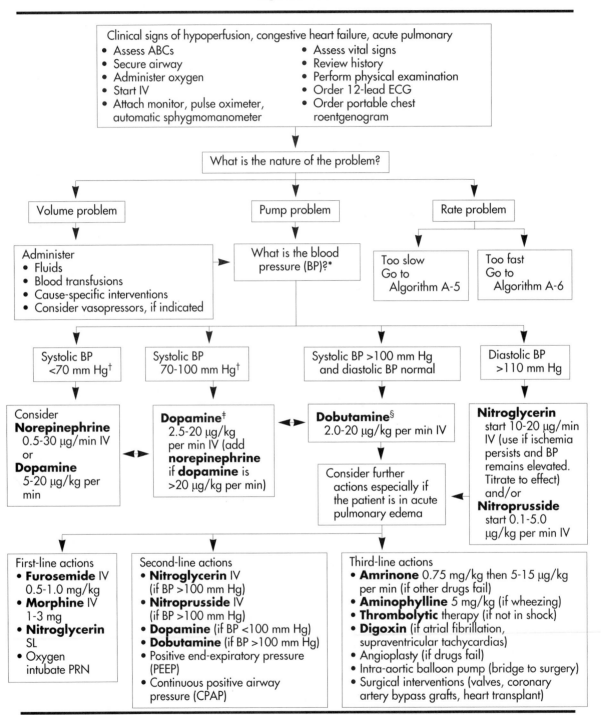

Clinical signs of hypoperfusion, congestive heart failure, acute pulmonary
- Assess ABCs
- Secure airway
- Administer oxygen
- Start IV
- Attach monitor, pulse oximeter, automatic sphygmomanometer
- Assess vital signs
- Review history
- Perform physical examination
- Order 12-lead ECG
- Order portable chest roentgenogram

What is the nature of the problem?

Volume problem | Pump problem | Rate problem

Administer
- Fluids
- Blood transfusions
- Cause-specific interventions
- Consider vasopressors, if indicated

What is the blood pressure (BP)?*

Too slow
Go to
Algorithm A-5

Too fast
Go to
Algorithm A-6

Systolic BP <70 mm Hg†

Systolic BP 70-100 mm Hg†

Systolic BP >100 mm Hg and diastolic BP normal

Diastolic BP >110 mm Hg

Consider
Norepinephrine 0.5-30 µg/min IV
or
Dopamine 5-20 µg/kg per min

Dopamine† 2.5-20 µg/kg per min IV (add **norepinephrine** if **dopamine** is >20 µg/kg per min)

Dobutamine§ 2.0-20 µg/kg per min IV

Consider further actions especially if the patient is in acute pulmonary edema

Nitroglycerin start 10-20 µg/min IV (use if ischemia persists and BP remains elevated. Titrate to effect) and/or
Nitroprusside start 0.1-5.0 µg/kg per min IV

First-line actions
- **Furosemide** IV 0.5-1.0 mg/kg
- **Morphine** IV 1-3 mg
- **Nitroglycerin** SL
- Oxygen intubate PRN

Second-line actions
- **Nitroglycerin** IV (if BP >100 mm Hg)
- **Nitroprusside** IV (if BP >100 mm Hg)
- **Dopamine** (if BP <100 mm Hg)
- **Dobutamine** (if BP >100 mm Hg)
- Positive end-expiratory pressure (PEEP)
- Continuous positive airway pressure (CPAP)

Third-line actions
- **Amrinone** 0.75 mg/kg then 5-15 µg/kg per min (if other drugs fail)
- **Aminophylline** 5 mg/kg (if wheezing)
- **Thrombolytic** therapy (if not in shock)
- **Digoxin** (if atrial fibrillation, supraventricular tachycardias)
- Angioplasty (if drugs fail)
- Intra-aortic balloon pump (bridge to surgery)
- Surgical interventions (valves, coronary artery bypass grafts, heart transplant)

Algorithm A-7   Algorithm for hypotension, shock, and acute pulmonary edema.

Algorithm A-7—*cont'd*

*Base management after this point on invasive hemodynamic monitoring if possible.

†Fluid bolus of 250-500 mL normal saline should be tried. If no response, consider sympathomimetics.

‡Move to **dopamine** and stop **norepinephrine** when BP improves.

§Add **dopamine** when BP improves. Avoid **dobutamine** when systolic BP <100 mm Hg.

Algorithm A-7—*cont'd.* (For legend see opposite page.)

Algorithm A-8

Community
- Community emphasis on "call first/call fast, call 9-1-1"
- National Heart Attack Alert Program

EMS System
EMS system approach that should address
- Oxygen-IV-cardiac monitor-vital signs
- **Nitroglycerin**
- Pain relief with narcotics
- Notification of emergency department
- Rapid transport to emergency department
- Prehospital screening for **thrombolytic therapy***
- 12-lead ECG, computer analysis, transmission to emergency department*
- Initiation of **thrombolytic therapy***

Emergency Department
"Door-to-drug" team protocol approach
- Rapid triage of patients with chest pain
- Clinical decision maker established
  (emergency physician, cardiologist, or other)

Time interval in emergency department

Assessment
Immediate:
- Vital signs with automatic BP
- Oxygen saturation
- Start IV
- 12-lead ECG (MD review)
- Brief, targeted history and physical
- Decide on eligibility for **thrombolytic** therapy

Soon:
- Chest roentgenogram
- Blood studies (electrolytes, enzymes, coagulation studies)
- Consult as needed

Treatments to consider if there is evidence of coronary thrombosis plus no reasons for exclusion (some but not all may be appropriate)
- Oxygen at 4 L/min
- **Nitroglycerin** SL, paste or spray (if systolic blood pressure >90 mm Hg)
- **Morphine** IV
- **Aspirin** PO
- **Thrombolytic** agents
- **Nitroglycerin** IV (limit systolic BP drop to 10% if normotensive; 30% drop if hypertensive; never drop below 90 mm Hg systolic)
- β-**blockers** IV
- **Heparin** IV
- Percutaneous transluminal coronary angioplasty
- Routine **lidocaine** administration is not recommended for all patients with AMI

30-60 min to **thrombolytic** therapy

*Optional guidelines

Algorithm A-8   Acute myocardial infarction (AMI) algorithm. Recommendations for early treatment of patients with chest pain and possible AMI.

B

Pediatric Advanced Life Support Guidelines

All the material contained in this appendix is reproduced with permission.

JAMA 1992; 268:2199-2275.

(See also "The Algorithm Approach to Emergency Cardiac Care" in Appendix A.)

Table B-1 Drugs Used in Pediatric Advanced Life Support

DRUGS	DOSE	REMARKS
Adenosine	0.1 to 0.2 mg/kg Maximum single dose: 12 mg	Rapid IV bolus
Atropine sulfate	0.02 mg/kg per dose	Minimum dose: 0.1 mg Maximum single dose: 0.5 mg in child, 1.0 mg in adolescent
Bretylium	5 mg/kg; may be increased to 10 mg/kg	Rapid IV
Calcium chloride 10%	20 mg/kg per dose	Give slowly
Dopamine hydrochloride	2-20 µg/kg per minute	α-Adrenergic action dominates at ≥15-20 µg/kg per minute
Dobutamine hydrochloride	2-20 µg/kg per minute	Titrate to desired effect
Epinephrine *For bradycardia*	IV/IO: 0.01 mg/kg (1:10,000) ET: 0.1 mg/kg (1:1000)	Be aware of effective dose of preservatives administered (if preservatives present in epinephrine preparation) when high doses are used
For asystolic or pulseless arrest	First dose: IV/IO: 0.01 mg/kg (1:10,000) ET: 0.1 mg/kg (1:1000) Doses as high as 0.2 mg/kg may be effective Subsequent doses: IV/IO/ET: 0.1 mg/kg (1:1000) Doses as high as 0.2 mg/kg may be effective	Be aware of effective dose of preservatives administered (if preservatives present in epinephrine preparation) when high doses are used
Epinephrine infusion	Initial at 0.1 µg/kg per minute Higher infusion dose used if asystole present	Titrate to desired effect (0.1-1.0 µg/kg per minute)
Lidocaine	1 mg/kg per dose	
Lidocaine infusion	20-50 µg/kg per dose	
Sodium bicarbonate	1 mEq/kg per dose or 0.3 × kg × base deficit	Infuse slowly and only if ventilation is adequate

IV, intravenous route; IO, intraosseous route; ET, endotracheal route.

Table B-2 Preparation of Infusions

DRUG	PREPARATION*	DOSE
Epinephrine	0.6 × body weight (kg) equals milligrams added to diluent[†] to make 100 mL	Then 1 mL/h delivers 0.1 µg/kg per minute; titrate to effect
Dopamine, dobutamine	6 × body weight (kg) equals milligrams added to diluent to make 100 mL	Then 1 mL/h delivers 1.0 µg/kg per minute; titrate to effect
Lidocaine	120 mg of 40-mg/mL solution added to 97 mL of 5% dextrose in water, yielding 1200 µg/mL solution	Then 1 mL/kg per hour delivers 20 µg/kg per minute

*Standard concentration may be used to provide more dilute or more concentrated drug solution, but then individual dose must be calculated for each patient and each infusion rate:

$$\text{Infusion rate (mL/h)} = \frac{\text{Weight (kg)} \times \text{Dose (µg/kg/min)} \times 60 \text{ min/h}}{\text{Concentration (µg/mL)}}$$

[†]Diluent may be 5% dextrose in water, 5% dextrose in half-normal saline, normal saline, or Ringer's lactate.

Algorithm B-1

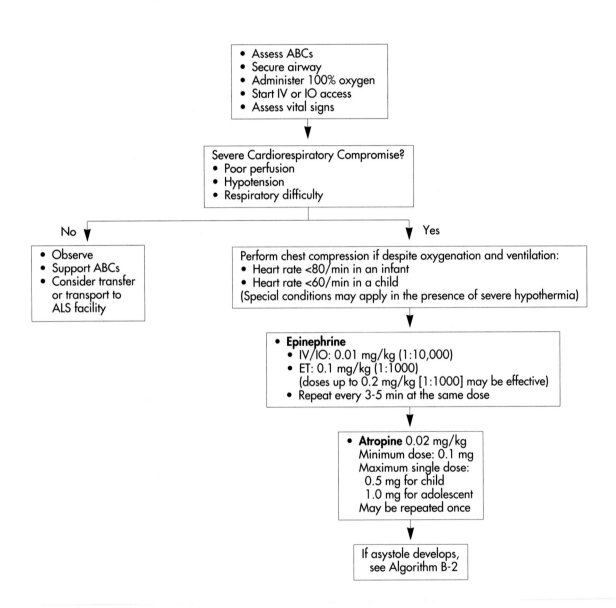

- Assess ABCs
- Secure airway
- Administer 100% oxygen
- Start IV or IO access
- Assess vital signs

Severe Cardiorespiratory Compromise?
- Poor perfusion
- Hypotension
- Respiratory difficulty

No

- Observe
- Support ABCs
- Consider transfer or transport to ALS facility

Yes

Perform chest compression if despite oxygenation and ventilation:
- Heart rate <80/min in an infant
- Heart rate <60/min in a child
(Special conditions may apply in the presence of severe hypothermia)

- **Epinephrine**
  - IV/IO: 0.01 mg/kg (1:10,000)
  - ET: 0.1 mg/kg (1:1000)
    (doses up to 0.2 mg/kg [1:1000] may be effective)
  - Repeat every 3-5 min at the same dose

- **Atropine** 0.02 mg/kg
  Minimum dose: 0.1 mg
  Maximum single dose:
  0.5 mg for child
  1.0 mg for adolescent
  May be repeated once

If asystole develops,
see Algorithm B-2

Algorithm B-1 Bradycardia decision tree. ABCs, airway, breathing, and circulation; ALS, advanced life support; ET, endotracheal; IO, intraosseous; IV, intravenous.

Algorithm B-2

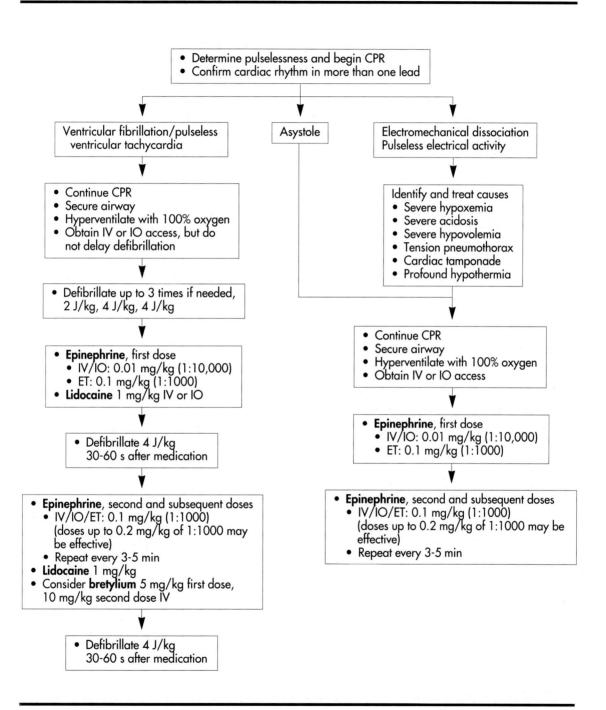

Algorithm B-2 Asystole and pulseless arrest decision tree. CPR, cardiopulmonary resuscitation; ET, endotracheal; IO, intraosseous; IV, intravenous.

C

Answers to Chapter 4 Self-tests

The following are the steps toward solving the conversion problems and the answers to the self-test on page 95:

1. x mg = 10 gr

$$= 10 \text{ gr} \times \frac{60 \text{ mg}}{1 \text{ gr}}$$

$$= 10 \text{ gr} \times \frac{60 \text{ mg}}{1 \text{ gr}}$$

$$= 600 \text{ mg}$$

2. x gr = 100 mg

$$= 100 \text{ mg} \times \frac{1 \text{ gr}}{60 \text{ mg}}$$

$$= 100 \text{ mg} \times \frac{1 \text{ gr}}{60 \text{ mg}}$$

$$= \frac{10}{6} \text{ gr} = 1.666 \text{ gr}$$

3. x mg = $\frac{1}{150}$ gr

$$= \frac{1}{150} \text{ gr} \times \frac{60 \text{ mg}}{1 \text{ gr}}$$

$$= \frac{1}{150} \text{ gr} \times \frac{60 \text{ mg}}{1 \text{ gr}}$$

$$= \frac{60 \text{ mg}}{150} = 0.4 \text{ mg}$$

4. x kg = 190 lb

$$= 190 \text{ lb} \times \frac{1 \text{ kg}}{2.2 \text{ lb}}$$

$$= 190 \text{ lb} \times \frac{1 \text{ kg}}{2.2 \text{ lb}}$$

$$= 86.36 \text{ kg}$$

5. x cm = 4 in

$$= 4 \text{ in} \times \frac{2.54 \text{ cm}}{1 \text{ in}}$$

$$= 4 \text{ in} \times \frac{2.54 \text{ cm}}{1 \text{ in}}$$

$$= 10.16 \text{ cm}$$

6. x lb = 40 kg

$$= 40 \text{ kg} \times \frac{2.2 \text{ lb}}{1 \text{ kg}}$$

$$= 40 \text{ kg} \times \frac{2.2 \text{ lb}}{1 \text{ kg}}$$

$$= 88 \text{ lb}$$

7. x mg = 3 g

$$= 3 \text{ g} \times \frac{1000 \text{ mg}}{1 \text{ g}}$$

$$= 3 \cancel{\text{g}} \times \frac{1000 \text{ mg}}{1 \cancel{\text{g}}}$$

$$= 3000 \text{ mg}$$

8. x liter = 500 ml

$$= 500 \text{ ml} \times \frac{1 \text{ liter}}{1000 \text{ ml}}$$

$$= 500 \cancel{\text{ml}} \times \frac{1 \text{ liter}}{1000 \cancel{\text{ml}}}$$

$$= 0.5 \text{ liter}$$

9. x mg = 1.5 kg

$$= 1.5 \text{ kg} \times \frac{1000 \text{ g}}{1 \text{ kg}} \times \frac{1000 \text{ mg}}{1 \text{ g}}$$

$$= 1.5 \cancel{\text{kg}} \times \frac{1000 \cancel{\text{g}}}{1 \cancel{\text{kg}}} \times \frac{1000 \text{ mg}}{1 \cancel{\text{g}}}$$

$$= 1,500,000 \text{ mg}$$

10. x g = 900 mg

$$= 900 \text{ mg} \times \frac{1 \text{ g}}{1000 \text{ mg}}$$

$$= 900 \cancel{\text{mg}} \times \frac{1 \text{ g}}{1000 \cancel{\text{mg}}}$$

$$= 0.9 \text{ g}$$

The following are the steps toward solving the calculation problems and the answers to the self-test on page 104:

1. Order: morphine sulfate 2 mg IV push.
   On hand: morphine sulfate 10 mg/ml. You dilute the morphine in 9 ml normal saline to equal 1 mg/ml. How many milliliters will you administer?

$$x \text{ ml} = \frac{1 \text{ ml}}{1 \text{ mg}} \times \frac{2 \text{ mg}}{1}$$

$$= \frac{1 \text{ ml}}{1 \cancel{\text{mg}}} \times \frac{2 \cancel{\text{mg}}}{1}$$

$$= \frac{1 \text{ ml} \times 2}{1}$$

$$= 2 \text{ ml}$$

2. Order: 12 mg adenosine IV push.
   On hand: adenosine 6 mg/2 ml. How many milliliters will you administer?

$$x \text{ ml} = \frac{2 \text{ ml}}{6 \text{ mg}} \times \frac{12 \text{ mg}}{1}$$

$$= \frac{2 \text{ ml}}{6 \cancel{\text{mg}}} \times \frac{12 \cancel{\text{mg}}}{1}$$

$$= \frac{2 \text{ ml} \times 2}{1}$$

$$= 4 \text{ ml}$$

3. Order: bretylium 5 mg/kg.
   On hand: bretylium 500 mg in 10 ml Patient weighs 242 lb.
   How many milliliters will you administer?

$$x \text{ ml} = \frac{10 \text{ ml}}{500 \text{ mg}} \times \frac{5 \text{ mg}}{\text{kg}} \times \frac{1 \text{ kg}}{2.2 \text{ lb}} \times \frac{242 \text{ lb}}{1}$$

$$= \frac{10 \text{ ml}}{500 \cancel{\text{mg}}} \times \frac{5 \cancel{\text{mg}}}{\cancel{\text{kg}}} \times \frac{1 \cancel{\text{kg}}}{2.2 \cancel{\text{lb}}} \times \frac{242 \cancel{\text{lb}}}{1}$$

$$= \frac{10 \text{ ml} \times 110}{100}$$

$$= 11 \text{ ml}$$

4. Order: epinephrine 1 µg/min.
   On hand: 1 mg diluted in 250 ml D₅W.
   Administration set delivers 60 gtts/ml.
   How many gtts/min will you deliver?

$$\frac{x \text{ gtts}}{\text{min}} = \frac{60 \text{ gtts}}{\text{ml}} \times \frac{250 \text{ ml}}{1 \text{ mg}} \times \frac{1 \text{ mg}}{1000 \text{ µg}} \times \frac{1 \text{ µg}}{\text{min}}$$

$$= \frac{60 \text{ gtts}}{\text{ml}} \times \frac{250 \text{ ml}}{1 \text{ mg}} \times \frac{1 \text{ mg}}{1000 \text{ µg}} \times \frac{1 \text{ µg}}{\text{min}}$$

$$= \frac{60 \text{ gtts} \times 1}{4 \text{ min}}$$

$$= \frac{15 \text{ gtts}}{\text{min}}$$

$$= 15 \text{ gtts/min}$$

5. Order: Demerol 35 mg IV push.
   On hand: Demerol 50 mg/ml.
   How many milliliters will you administer?

$$x \text{ ml} = \frac{1 \text{ ml}}{50 \text{ mg}} \times \frac{35 \text{ mg}}{1}$$

$$= \frac{1 \text{ ml}}{50 \text{ mg}} \times \frac{35 \text{ mg}}{1}$$

$$= \frac{7 \text{ ml}}{10}$$

$$= 0.7 \text{ ml}$$

6. Order: oxytocin 5 units IM.
   On hand: oxytocin 10 units/ml.
   How many milliliters will you administer?

$$x \text{ ml} = \frac{1 \text{ ml}}{10 \text{ units}} \times \frac{5 \text{ units}}{1}$$

$$= \frac{1 \text{ ml}}{10 \text{ units}} \times \frac{5 \text{ units}}{1}$$

$$= \frac{1 \text{ ml}}{2}$$

$$= 0.5 \text{ ml}$$

7. Order: Ringer's lactate 300 ml over 30 min.
   On hand: Ringer's lactate 1000 ml.

Administration set delivers 10 gtts/ml.
How many gtts/min will you administer?

$$\frac{x \text{ gtts}}{\text{min}} = \frac{10 \text{ gtts}}{\text{ml}} \times \frac{300 \text{ ml}}{30 \text{ min}}$$

$$= \frac{10 \text{ gtts}}{\text{ml}} \times \frac{300 \text{ ml}}{30 \text{ min}}$$

$$= \frac{10 \text{ gtts} \times 10}{1 \text{ min}}$$

$$= \frac{100 \text{ gtts}}{\text{min}}$$

$$= 100 \text{ gtts/min}$$

8. Order: furosemide 60 mg IV push.
   On hand: furosemide 20 mg/2 ml.
   How many milliliters will you administer?

$$x \text{ ml} = \frac{2 \text{ ml}}{20 \text{ mg}} \times \frac{60 \text{ mg}}{1}$$

$$= \frac{2 \text{ ml}}{20 \text{ mg}} \times \frac{60 \text{ mg}}{1}$$

$$= \frac{6 \text{ ml}}{1}$$

$$= 6 \text{ ml}$$

9. Order: atropine 0.5 mg IV push.
   On hand: atropine 1 mg/ml.
   How many milliliters will you administer?

$$x \text{ ml} = \frac{1 \text{ ml}}{1 \text{ mg}} \times \frac{0.5 \text{ mg}}{1}$$

$$= \frac{1 \text{ ml}}{1 \text{ mg}} \times \frac{0.5 \text{ mg}}{1}$$

$$= 0.5 \text{ ml}$$

10. Order: isoproterenol 4 µg/min via IV infusion.
    On hand: 1 mg isoproterenol per 250 ml D$_5$W.
    Administration set delivers 60 gtts/ml.
    How many gtts/min will you administer?

$$\frac{x \text{ gtts}}{\text{min}} = \frac{60 \text{ gtts}}{\text{ml}} \times \frac{250 \text{ ml}}{1 \text{ mg}} \times \frac{1 \text{ mg}}{1000 \text{ µg}} \times \frac{4 \text{ µg}}{\text{min}}$$

$$= \frac{60 \text{ gtts}}{\text{ml}} \times \frac{250 \text{ ml}}{1 \text{ mg}} \times \frac{1 \text{ mg}}{1000 \text{ µg}} \times \frac{4 \text{ µg}}{\text{min}}$$

$$= \frac{60 \text{ gtts} \times 4}{4 \text{ min}}$$

$$= 60 \text{ gtts/min}$$

11. Order: normal saline 1000 ml over 4 hours.
    On hand: normal saline 1000 ml and administration set, which delivers 15 gtts/ml.
    How many gtts/min will you administer?

$$\frac{x \text{ gtts}}{\text{min}} = \frac{15 \text{ gtts}}{\text{ml}} \times \frac{1000 \text{ ml}}{4 \text{ hr}} \times \frac{1 \text{ hr}}{60 \text{ min}}$$

$$= \frac{15 \text{ gtts}}{\text{ml}} \times \frac{1000 \text{ ml}}{4 \text{ hr}} \times \frac{1 \text{ hr}}{60 \text{ min}}$$

$$= \frac{15 \text{ gtts} \times 250}{60 \text{ min}}$$

$$= \frac{62.5 \text{ gtts}}{\text{min}}$$

$$= \text{round to } 63 \text{ gtts/min}$$

12. Order: dobutamine 8 µg/kg/min via IV infusion.
    On hand: dobutamine 250 mg in 250 ml D$_5$W.
    Administration set delivers 60 gtts/ml.
    Patient weighs 198 lbs.
    How many ml/hr will the patient receive?

$$\frac{x \text{ ml}}{\text{min}} = \frac{250 \text{ ml}}{250 \text{ mg}} \times \frac{1 \text{ mg}}{1000 \text{ µg}} \times \frac{8 \text{ µg}}{\text{kg min}} \times \frac{1 \text{ kg}}{2.2 \text{ lb}} \times \frac{198 \text{ lb}}{1} \times \frac{60 \text{ min}}{1 \text{ hr}}$$

$$= \frac{250 \text{ ml}}{250 \text{ mg}} \times \frac{1 \text{ mg}}{1000 \text{ µg}} \times \frac{8 \text{ µg}}{\text{kg min}} \times \frac{1 \text{ kg}}{2.2 \text{ lb}} \times \frac{198 \text{ lb}}{1} \times \frac{60 \text{ min}}{1 \text{ hr}}$$

$$= \frac{4 \text{ ml} \times 90 \times 60}{500 \text{ hr}}$$

$$= \frac{43.2 \text{ ml}}{\text{hr}}$$

$$= \text{round to } 43 \text{ ml/hr}$$

13. Order: dopamine 6 µg/kg/min via IV infusion.
    On hand: dopamine 400 mg in 500 ml D$_5$W.
    Administration set delivers 60 gtts/ml.
    Patient weighs 90 kg.
    Determine the rate of infusion in gtts/min.

$$\frac{x \text{ gtts}}{\text{min}} = \frac{60 \text{ gtts}}{\text{ml}} \times \frac{500 \text{ ml}}{400 \text{ mg}} \times \frac{1 \text{ mg}}{1000 \text{ μg}} \times \frac{6 \text{ μg}}{\text{kg min}} \times \frac{90 \text{ kg}}{1}$$

$$= \frac{60 \text{ gtts}}{\text{ml}} \times \frac{500 \text{ ml}}{400 \text{ mg}} \times \frac{1 \text{ mg}}{1000 \text{ μg}} \times \frac{6 \text{ μg}}{\text{kg min}} \times \frac{90 \text{ kg}}{1}$$

$$= \frac{6 \text{ gtts} \times 6 \times 90}{40 \times 2 \text{ min}}$$

$$= \frac{3240 \text{ gtts}}{80 \text{ min}}$$

$$= \frac{40.5 \text{ gtts}}{\text{min}}$$

$$= \text{round to 41 gtts/min}$$

14. Order: lidocaine 2 mg/min via IV infusion.
    On hand: lidocaine 2 g in 500 ml D_5W.
    How many ml/hr will you administer?

$$\frac{x \text{ ml}}{\text{hr}} = \frac{500 \text{ ml}}{2 \text{ g}} \times \frac{1 \text{ g}}{1000 \text{ mg}} \times \frac{2 \text{ mg}}{\text{min}} \times \frac{60 \text{ min}}{\text{hr}}$$

$$= \frac{500 \text{ ml}}{2 \text{ g}} \times \frac{1 \text{ g}}{1000 \text{ mg}} \times \frac{2 \text{ mg}}{\text{min}} \times \frac{60 \text{ min}}{\text{hr}}$$

$$= \frac{2 \times 60 \text{ ml}}{2 \times 2 \text{ hr}}$$

$$= \frac{30 \text{ ml}}{\text{hr}}$$

$$= 30 \text{ ml/hr}$$

15. Order: Ringer's lactate 250 ml over 90 min.
    On hand: Ringer's lactate, 500 ml.
    Administration set delivers 20 gtts/ml.
    How many gtts/min will you deliver?

$$\frac{x \text{ gtts}}{\text{min}} = \frac{20 \text{ gtts}}{\text{ml}} \times \frac{250 \text{ ml}}{90 \text{ min}}$$

$$= \frac{20 \text{ gtts}}{\text{ml}} \times \frac{250 \text{ ml}}{90 \text{ min}}$$

$$= \frac{2 \times 250 \text{ gtts}}{9 \text{ min}}$$

$$= \frac{55.5 \text{ gtts}}{\text{min}}$$

$$= \text{round to } 56 \text{ gtts/min}$$

16. Patient is receiving nitroprusside via IV infusion at 1 μg/kg/min. The order is to reduce the rate of infusion to 0.8 μg/kg/min. The concentration of the solution is 200 μg/ml. The patient weighs 220 lb. The solution set provides 60 gtts/ml. What is the new rate in gtts/min?

$$\frac{x \text{ gtts}}{\text{min}} = \frac{60 \text{ gtts}}{\text{ml}} \times \frac{1 \text{ ml}}{200 \text{ μg}} \times \frac{0.8 \text{ μg}}{\text{kg min}} \times \frac{1 \text{ kg}}{2.2 \text{ lb}} \times \frac{220 \text{ lb}}{1}$$

$$= \frac{60 \text{ gtts}}{\text{ml}} \times \frac{1 \text{ ml}}{200 \text{ μg}} \times \frac{0.8 \text{ μg}}{\text{kg min}} \times \frac{1 \text{ kg}}{2.2 \text{ lb}} \times \frac{220 \text{ lb}}{1}$$

$$= \frac{6 \times 0.8 \times 100 \text{ gtts}}{20 \times 1 \text{ min}}$$

$$= \frac{24 \text{ gtts}}{\text{min}}$$

$$= 24 \text{ gtts/min}$$

17. The patient is receiving dopamine at a rate of 25 ml/hr. The concentration of the solution is 200 mg in 250 ml D$_5$W.
    How many μg/kg/min is this 90 kg person receiving?

$$\frac{x \text{ μg}}{\text{kg min}} = \frac{1000 \text{ μg}}{1 \text{ mg}} \times \frac{200 \text{ mg}}{250 \text{ ml}} \times \frac{25 \text{ ml}}{1 \text{ hr}} \times \frac{1 \text{ hr}}{60 \text{ min}} \times \frac{1}{90 \text{ kg}}$$

$$= \frac{1000 \text{ μg}}{1 \text{ mg}} \times \frac{200 \text{ mg}}{250 \text{ ml}} \times \frac{25 \text{ ml}}{1 \text{ hr}} \times \frac{1 \text{ hr}}{60 \text{ min}} \times \frac{1}{90 \text{ kg}}$$

$$= \frac{4 \times 20 \times 25 \text{ μg}}{6 \times 90 \text{ kg min}}$$

$$= \frac{2000 \text{ μg}}{540 \text{ kg min}}$$

$$= \frac{3.7 \text{ μg}}{\text{kg min}}$$

$$= 3.7 \text{ μg/kg/min}$$

18. The patient is receiving aminophylline via IV infusion at 100 ml/30 min. The concentration of the solution is 125 mg aminophylline in 100 ml D$_5$W.
    How many mg/min is the patient receiving?

$$\frac{x \text{ mg}}{\text{min}} = \frac{125 \text{ mg}}{100 \text{ ml}} \times \frac{100 \text{ ml}}{30 \text{ min}}$$

$$= \frac{125 \text{ mg}}{100 \text{ ml}} \times \frac{100 \text{ ml}}{30 \text{ min}}$$

$$= \frac{125 \text{ mg}}{30 \text{ min}}$$

$$= 4.16 \text{ mg/min}$$

$$= \text{round to } 4 \text{ mg/min}$$

19. The patient is receiving morphine sulfate via IV infusion. The concentration of the solution is 100 mg morphine sulfate in 500 ml IV fluid. It is infusing at a rate of 30 ml/hr.

    How many mg/hr is the patient receiving?

$$\frac{x \text{ mg}}{\text{hr}} = \frac{100 \text{ mg}}{500 \text{ ml}} \times \frac{30 \text{ ml}}{1 \text{ hr}}$$

$$= \frac{100 \text{ mg}}{500 \text{ ml}} \times \frac{30 \text{ ml}}{1 \text{ hr}}$$

$$= \frac{30 \text{ mg}}{5 \text{ hr}}$$

$$= \frac{6 \text{ mg}}{\text{hr}}$$

$$= 6 \text{ mg/hr}$$

20. Your patient is receiving a lidocaine drip at 45 gtts/min. The label indicates that 2 g of lidocaine were added to 500 ml D$_5$W.

    How many mg/min is the patient receiving? (Administration set = 60 drops/ml)

$$\frac{x \text{ mg}}{\text{min}} = \frac{1000 \text{ mg}}{\text{g}} \times \frac{2 \text{ g}}{500 \text{ ml}} \times \frac{1 \text{ ml}}{60 \text{ gtts}} \times \frac{45 \text{ gtts}}{\text{min}}$$

$$= \frac{1000 \text{ mg}}{\text{g}} \times \frac{2 \text{ g}}{500 \text{ ml}} \times \frac{1 \text{ ml}}{60 \text{ gtts}} \times \frac{45 \text{ gtts}}{\text{min}}$$

$$= \frac{2 \times 45 \text{ gtts}}{30 \text{ min}}$$

$$= \frac{3 \text{ mg}}{\text{min}}$$

$$= 3 \text{ mg/min}$$

Glossary

Absolute refractory absolute refractory refers to that interval of time following depolarization during which the cell is incapable of responding to another stimulus.

Absorption the process by which a drug moves from its site of entry into the body and into circulating fluids for distribution.

Acetylcholine a neurotransmitter in all autonomic preganglionic synapses.

Active transport the movement of substances against a concentration gradient.

Additive the sum of the effects of two drugs.

Adrenal medulla a secretary organ located atop the kidney that manufactures and secretes epinephrine and norepinephrine.

Adrenergic of or pertaining to sympathetic nerve fibers.

Adsorbent a substance that holds a gas or soluble substance on its surface.

Adverse reaction undesirable or potentially harmful side effects of a drug.

Affinity the tendency or propensity of a drug to combine with a specific receptor site.

Afterload the pressure against which the ventricle has to contract to eject its contents; increased arterial pressure increases afterload.

Agonist a drug that combines with a receptor to elicit a physiologic response.

Analgesic a drug that relieves pain.

Anion a negatively charged ion.

Antagonism when one drug interferes with or reduces the effects of another.

Antecubital veins the portion of the basilic and cephalic vein located in the antecubital fossa (the bend of the elbow).

Antidote a substance that neutralizes poisons or their effects.

Atherosclerosis an arterial disorder characterized by plaques of cholesterol, lipids, and cellular debris in the inner layers of the artery walls.

Automaticity the property of the cells of the heart's conducting system whereby an impulse is initiated without outside stimulation; self-excitation or self-depolarization.

Axon an extension of a nerve cell that carries impulses away from the nerve cell body.

Benzodiazepine a group of psychotropic drugs used primarily to treat anxiety and to induce sleep.

Binding capacity the degree to which a drug is bound to tissue or plasma proteins at any given time.

Biotransformation (see metabolism).

Bolus a method of intravenous medication administration by which a drug is rapidly administered rather than infuse over a period of time.

Bronchospasm contraction of the smooth muscle of the bronchioles, resulting in acute narrowing of the airway lumen and obstruction to air flow; characterized by generalized wheezing.

Buccal pertaining to the inside of the cheek; a route of medication administration by which a drug is absorbed across the mucous membranes of the cheek and gums.

Cannulation the insertion of a cannula into a blood vessel.

Capillary blood glucose measuring devices devices used to measure blood sugar; a drop of blood is placed on a reagent strip or cartridge; the blood glucose level is displayed digitally.

Cardiac output (CO) the volume of blood pumped by the heart per minute (about 5 liters in average adult); cardiac output is a function of stroke volume and heart rate (HR) and is represented by the formula $SV \times HR = CO$.

Cation a positively charged ion.

Chemical name the name that describes the chemical composition and molecular structure of a drug.

Cholinergic of or pertaining to nerve fibers that synthesize acetylcholine.

Chronic obstructive pulmonary disease (COPD) a progressive condition characterized by diminished ventilatory function; includes emphysema, bronchitis, and asthma.

Chronotropic an adjective that refers to a drug's effect on heart rate; when a drug is said to have a positive chronotropic effect it results in an increase in heart rate; a negative chronotropic effect refers to a decrease in heart rate.

Clonic the phase of a seizure characterized by alternating contraction and relaxation of muscles.

Colloid osmotic pressure pressure generated by the presence of colloids in a solution.

Colloids substance of high molecular weight, such as plasma proteins.

Coma a state of deep unconsciousness in which the patient cannot be awakened and is not responsive to verbal and painful stimuli.

Conduction the transmission of impulses from one cardiac cell to another.

Conduction velocity the speed with which impulses are transmitted from one cell to another.

Conversion factor an equivalent numeric value that produces a change in the form of a quantity without changing its value.

Crystalloid a solution containing crystalline substances, such as normal saline.

Cumulative effect drug effects that develop when a dose is repeated before prior dose is metabolized. Drugs are accumulated and eventually produce symptoms of toxicity.

Dead space that portion of the airway in which gas exchange does not take place; anatomic dead space includes the trachea, bronchi, and bronchioles.

Decontamination the removal or neutralization of a poison.

Denominator divisor; the term of a fraction that expresses the number of equal parts into which a unit is divided; the denominator appears below or to the right of the line.

Depolarization   the process by which cardiac contraction is initiated; it is accomplished by the movement of electrolytes across the cell membrane and a change in the electrical charge of the cell membrane.

Depressant   a drug that diminishes the activity of the body or any of its organs.

Diabetes mellitus   a complex disorder of carbohydrate, fat, and protein metabolism in which there is an absolute or relative lack of insulin.

Diffusion   the movement of solutes from an area of high concentration to an area of lower concentration.

Dissolution   the process by which a solid form of a drug becomes soluble in body fluids.

Distribution   the process by which a drug is carried from its site of absorption to its site of action.

Dromotropic   an adjective that refers to a drug's effect on conduction velocity; a positive dromotropic effect refers to an increase in conduction velocity; a negative dromotropic effect refers to a decrease in conduction velocity.

Drug   any chemical that affects living processes.

Drug interaction   the process by which the expected therapeutic effect of a drug is altered by the introduction of another drug.

Effector organ   an organ or group of tissues on which the autonomic nervous system exerts an effect; target organ.

Elimination   (see excretion).

Emetic   a therapeutic agent that induces vomiting.

Endotracheal   within the trachea, a route of medication administration by which drugs are administered down an endotracheal tube.

Enteral   via the gastrointestinal tract.

Exacerbate   to aggravate symptoms or increase the severity of a disease.

Exacerbation   an increase in the severity of a disease.

Excessive postpartum bleeding   blood loss of 500 ml or more, resulting in hypovolemia; also referred to as postpartum hemorrhage.

Excitability   the ability of a cell to respond to an electrical stimulus.

Excretion (elimination)   the removal of drugs from the body via urine, bile, sweat, saliva, breast milk, and expired air.

Extracellular   outside of the cell wall.

Filtration   the movement of fluid and electrolytes in response to hydrostatic pressure.

Ganglia   a mass of nerve cells.

Generic name   the name that is often related to the chemical name of a drug but is completely independent of the manufacturer(s); the nonproprietary designation of a drug.

Habituation   psychological or emotional dependence on a drug after repeated use.

Half-life   the amount of time required to reduce the concentration of a drug in the blood by 50%.

Hydrostatic pressure   the pressure exerted by a fluid.

Hypercarbia   hypercapnia; too much carbon dioxide in the blood.

Hyperglycemia   a blood glucose level above normal; most often associated with diabetes mellitus.

Hypersensitivity   an exaggerated response to a drug, usually idiosyncratic in origin.

Hypertonic   having a solute concentration greater than that of another solution.

Hypoglycemia a blood glucose level below normal, usually related to the administration of too much insulin, excessive production of insulin by the pancreas, or inadequate dietary intake.

Hypotonic having a lesser solute concentration than that of another solution.

Hypoxia inadequate tissue oxygenation; reduced tension of cellular oxygen.

Idiosyncracy abnormal, unpredictable response to a drug peculiar to an individual.

Inhalation a route of medication administration by which drugs in the form of a fine mist or spray are inhaled.

Inotropic an adjective that refers to a drug's effect on the heart's force of contraction; when a drug is said to have a positive inotropic effect it results in an increased force of contraction; a negative inotropic effect refers to a decrease in the force of contraction.

Insidious of or pertaining to a gradual or imperceptible onset.

Insulin-dependent diabetes mellitus (IDDM) Type I diabetes mellitus in which there is no insulin production by the beta cells of the pancreas; patients with IDDM are dependent on insulin injections for survival.

Intracardiac within the heart.

Intracellular within the cell wall.

Intradermal a parenteral route of medication administration by which a drug is injected into the dermal layer of the skin.

Intramuscular within the muscle; a common parenteral route of medication administration by which a drug is injected into skeletal muscle.

Intraosseous a route of medication administration by which a drug is administered in the medullary canal of a long bone.

Intravascular within the blood vessels.

Intravenous within the vein; a commonly used parenteral route of medication administration by which a drug is injected directly into venous circulation.

Isotonic having the same solute concentration as another solution.

Ketones normal metabolic products (β-hydroxybutyric acid); excessive production of these occurs in uncontrolled diabetes mellitus.

Mechanism of action the way by which a drug produces its desired effect.

Metabolism (biotransformation) the process by which a drug is converted to a compound that can be excreted from the body.

Metered-dose inhaler a device for administering medications by inhalation; it consists of a canister containing a liquid that when activated delivers the medication in a fine mist.

Milliequivalent the concentration of electrolytes in a specific volume of solution; serum electrolytes are usually reported in terms of milliequivalents per liter.

Monosaccharide a simple sugar, such as glucose, fructose, or galactose.

Nebulizer a device that delivers liquid medication in a fine spray; nebulizers are usually powered by oxygen or compressed air.

Neurotransmitter a chemical substance that, when released, transmits impulses across a synapse.

Noninsulin-dependent diabetes mellitus (NIDDM) Type II diabetes mellitus in which there is insufficient production of insulin by the beta cells of the pancreas or resistance to the effects of insulin by the cells of the body; patients with NIDDM are managed by diet, exercise, and oral hypoglycemic agents; insulin injections are required by some NIDDM patients.

Norepinephrine a sympathetic neurotransmitter; the neurotransmitter in most postganglionic sympathetic synapses.

Numerator the term of a fraction above or to the left of the line that expresses the number of parts of a unit.

Opioid a group of synthetic narcotics not derived from opium.

Osmosis the movement of water or other solvents across a semipermeable membrane from an area of low solute concentration to an area of high solute concentration.

Parenteral occuring outside of the gastrointestinal tract; any route of medication administration that bypasses the gastrointestinal tract.

Passive transport the transport of fluid and/or electrolytes without energy expenditure; three means of active transport are diffusion, filtration, and osmosis.

pH the negative log of hydrogen ion concentration; a measure of the acidity or alkalinity of a substance.

Pharmacodynamics the study of the way drugs act on living tissues.

Pharmacokinetics the fate of drugs in the body, including absorption, distribution, metabolism, and excretion.

Pharmacology the study of drugs and their interactions with living systems.

Phlebitis inflammation of a vein.

Poison any substance that interferes with normal physiologic functions; most substances can be poisonous if consumed in sufficient quantity; poison implies an excessive dosage rather than a group of substances.

Polydipsia excessive thirst.

Polyuria excessive urinary output.

Postganglionic axon the axon that conducts impulses from the spinal cord to the ganglia.

Preload the amount (volume) of blood in the ventricle at the end of diastole; as venous return increases preload increases; increased preload is accompanied by increased stretch on the myocardial muscle resulting in increased force of contraction in the normal heart.

Protocols specified treatment regimens, standing orders.

Reagent a substance that detects the presence of another substance; glucose reagent strips detect the presence of glucose in blood; the glucose level is indicated by change in color.

Rectal via the rectum; an enteral route of medication administration by which the drug is instilled in the rectal vault.

Relative refractory relative refractory is that period of time during which a stronger stimulus than normal is required to elicit a response.

Renin an enzyme that affects blood pressure by catalyzing angiotensinogen to angiotensin, a strong pressor.

Repolarization return of the cell to its resting state.

Seizure a sudden, involuntary series of contractions of a group of muscles.

Shock inadequate tissue perfusion characterized by cellular dysfunction, hypotension, and oliguria.

Side effect   an effect of a drug other than that which is desired.

SLUDGE   a mnemonic for recognizing the signs and symptoms of organophosphate poisoning (salivation, lacrimation, urination, defecation, gastrointestinal distress, and emesis).

Slurry   a diluted, watery mixture.

Solute   a substance or particle dissolved in a solution.

Stat   immediately.

Status epilepticus   continual attacks of tonic-clonic seizure activity without intervals of consciousness.

Stimulant   a drug that increases the activity of the body or any of its organs.

Stroke volume (SV)   the amount of blood ejected by the ventricle with each contraction.

Subcutaneous   beneath the skin; a common parenteral route of medication administration by which a drug is injected into the loose connective tissue between the dermis and the muscle.

Sublingual   beneath the tongue; a route of medication administration by which a drug is absorbed across the rich blood supply of the inferior surface of the tongue.

Synapse   the junction between two nerve cells or between a nerve cell and an effector organ.

Synergism   an enhanced response resulting from concurrent use of two or more drugs.

Thromboembolism   the obstruction of a blood vessel by a thrombus that is detached from its site.

Thrombophlebitis   inflammation of a vein associated with clot formation.

Tidal volume   the amount of air inhaled and exhaled during normal ventilation.

Titrate   to adjust the administration rate of a medication in response to the effect on specific physiologic parameters, such as pulse or blood pressure.

Tolerance   decreased response to a drug with repeated doses.

Tonic   referring to a major motor seizure; the phase of a seizure characterized by a rigid contraction/tension of muscles.

Tonicity   the effect exerted by the osmolality of a solution.

Toxemia   distribution of poisonous products of bacteria throughout the body.

Toxicity   the degree to which a substance is poisonous.

Trade name   the name given a drug by its manufacturer; brand name; proprietary name.

Transdermal   across the skin; a route of medication administration used when slow absorption is acceptable or desirable.

Universal precautions   infection control procedures applicable to all patients.

Uterine atony   lack of normal tone or strength of the uterus.

Vasomotor   of or pertaining to the nerves or muscles that control the lumen of the blood vessel.

Venipuncture   the insertion of a needle or catheter through the skin into a vein for the purpose of administering fluid or drugs or for obtaining a blood specimen.

Ventilation   the process by which air is moved in and out of the lungs.

Wernicke-Korsakoff's syndrome   encephalopathy caused by a thiamine deficiency and seen with chronic alcoholism, may be mild or severe and is characterized by decreased mental function, lack of muscle coordination, involuntary rapid movement of the eyes, and double vision.

Index

Other Mosby Texts of Interest

BOOK CODE	AUTHOR/TITLE	PUBLICATION DATE
21764	ACLS: Video Series	12/91
00200	Allison: Advanced Life Support Skills	8/93
07067	American Red Cross CPR for the Professional Rescuer Text	3/93
21231	American Red Cross Emergency Response Text	3/93
07405	American Safety Video Publishers: Learning ECGs Video Series	10/93
00258	Atwood: Introduction to Cardiac Dysrhythmias	3/90
00385	Auf der Heide: Disaster Response	6/89
01185	Bosker: The 60-Second EMT	11/87
01330	Bronstein: Emergency Care for Hazardous Materials Exposure	5/88
01458	doCarmo: Basic EMT Skills and Equipment	8/88
01969	Gonsoulin: Prehospital Drug Therapy	9/93
02410	Huszar: Basic Dysrhythmia Interpretation and Management	7/88
02927	Huszar: Early Defibrillation	6/91
03353	Judd: First Responder: Textbook/ Workbook Package, 2/e	10/88
08077	Kidd: Engine Company: 1st Due Video Series	12/93
08093	Kidd: Rescue Company: 1st Due Video Series	12/93
06195	Krebs: When Violence Erupts	4/90
05853	Mack: EMT Certification Preparation	2/90
03375	Madigan: Prehospital Emergency Drugs Pocket Reference	3/90

BOOK CODE	AUTHOR/TITLE	PUBLICATION DATE
05791	Miller: Manual of Prehospital Emergency Medicine	3/92
03351	Moore: Vehicle Rescue and Extrication	9/90
05854	NAEMSP/Kuehl: EMS Medical Directors' Handbook	8/89
06579	NAEMSP/Swor: Quality Management in Prehospital Care	1/93
04284	Rothenberg: Advanced Medical Life Support	11/87
04894	Simon: Pediatric Life Support	11/88
05321	Ward: Prehospital Treatment Protocols	3/89
03525	Yvorra: Mosby's Emergency Dictionary	10/88

FOR ORDERING INFORMATION, CALL 1-800-426-4545

FREE ISSUE

Finally . . . see what you've been missing! Order a **FREE** issue of
JEMS, <u>the</u> premier EMS journal, today!

☐ **What a deal!** Send me a free issue of *JEMS* to look over. If I
decide to subscribe, I'll pay just $21.97 (over 20% off the regular
price) for 12 more issues (a one-year subscription).

Name _____

Title _____

Organization _____

Address _____

City _____ State _____ Zip_____

Please allow 2-8 weeks for your issue to arrive.

Important:

Please indicate Occupation/ Position
(Check one box only)

☐ A. Physician
☐ B. Nurse/Inst./Coord.
☐ C. Administrator/Supervisor
☐ D. Paramedic/EMT-1/EMT-D
☐ E. EMT (Basic, 1st Responder)
☐ F. Other _____
(Please Specify)

Please indicate Employer/ Affiliation
(Check one box only)

☐ 1. Hospital
☐ 2. Private Ambulance
☐ 3. Fire Dept./Rescue Squad
☐ 4. Third Serv./Mun. Agency
☐ 5. Industrial/Commercial
☐ 6. Other _____
(Please Specify)

338ZV

SAMPLE COPY

Prehospital and Disaster Medicine

☐ **Yes!** Send me a no-obligation sample copy of
Prehospital and Disaster Medicine, FREE.

If I like what I see, I'll pay just $29 for a full year subscription and get 3 more journals
(4 in all). If I'm not satisfied I'll just write 'cancel' on the bill and return it.

Name _____

Title _____

Organization _____

Address _____

City _____ State_____ Zip_____

338ZX

Please Indicate Your Occupation:

☐ Physician
☐ Nurse
☐ EMT/Paramedic
☐ Administrative/Supv./Purch. Agent
☐ Disaster/Civil Defense Planner
☐ Other_____

Please Indicate Your Employment Location:

☐ Hospital
☐ Fire Dept./Rescue Squad
☐ Ambulance Service
☐ Regional/State/Fed Agency
☐ Industry
☐ Other _____

Please Indicate Your PRIMARY SPECIALTY (if Physician):

☐ Emergency Medicine
☐ Critical Care
☐ Traumatology
☐ Prehospital Medical Director
☐ Cardiology
☐ Other _____

Allow 2–6 weeks for your issue to be shipped

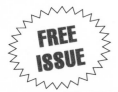

FREE ISSUE

BUSINESS REPLY MAIL
FIRST CLASS MAIL   PERMIT NO. 806   CARLSBAD, CA

POSTAGE WILL BE PAID BY ADDRESSEE

jems

PO BOX 469010
ESCONDIDO CA 92046-9976

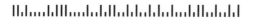

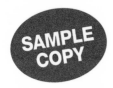

SAMPLE COPY

BUSINESS REPLY MAIL
FIRST CLASS MAIL   PERMIT NO. 759   CARLSBAD, CA

POSTAGE WILL BE PAID BY ADDRESSEE

PDM
PREHOSPITAL and
DISASTER MEDICINE
PO BOX 2789
CARLSBAD CA 92018-9898

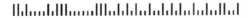